S. Dithmar

F.G. Holz

Fluorescence Angiography in Ophthalmology

S. Dithmar

F.G. Holz

Fluorescence Angiography in Ophthalmology

With 541 Figures

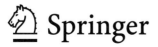
Springer

Prof. Dr. Stefan Dithmar, MD
Section of Vitreoretinal Surgery & Disease
Department of Ophthalmology
University of Heidelberg
Im Neuenheimer Feld 400
69120 Heidelberg
Germany

Prof. Dr. Frank G. Holz, MD
Chair of the Department of Ophthalmology
University of Bonn
Ernst-Abbe-Str.2
53127 Bonn
Germany

Translation:
William M Hart, MD, Ph.D.
Professor
Department of Ophthalmology and Visual
Sciences
Washington University School of Medicine
St. Louis, MO 63110
USA

ISBN 978-3-540-78359-6 Springer Medizin Verlag Heidelberg

Bibliografische Information der Deutschen Bibliothek
The Deutsche Bibliothek lists this publication in Deutsche Nationalbibliographie;
detailed bibliographic data is available in the internet at http://dnb.ddb.de.

Springer Medizin Verlag
springer.com
© Springer Medizin Verlag Heidelberg 2008

Planning: Hanna Hensler-Fritton, Heidelberg
Project management: Barbara Knüchel, Heidelberg
Design: deblik Berlin
Translated by Prof. Dr. William Hart from the German edition: Fluoreszenzangiographie in der Augenheilkunde
    edited by S. Dithmar and F. Holz. 2007
Typesetting: TypoStudio Tobias Schaedla, Heidelberg

SPIN: 12232789

Gedruckt auf säurefreiem Papier   5135 – 5 4 3 2

Preface

Fluorescein and Indocyanine green angiography, including the imaging of fundus autofluorescence, has been significantly improved in the last few years. The use of confocal laser technology in particular has been the most significant improvement: the technology is digital, fluorescein and indocyanine green angiography are seen in real time and can be used simultaneously. The clinical findings have been expanded with the addition of infrared, red-free and autofluorescence imaging. The foundations for the new fluorescence angiography atlas of Professor S. Dithmar, Heidelberg and Professor F. Holz (previously of Heidelberg) are findings that have been gathered at the Heidelberg University Department of Ophthalmology with the Heidelberg Angiograph 2 (HRA 2, Heidelberg Engineering. This work documents the authors' successful collaboration with the Heidelberg Engineering firm.

This atlas clearly explains the technical fundamentals of fluorescence angiography and the imaging of pathological fluorescence phenomena. A full chapter is devoted to fundus autofluorescence, particularly with regard to pathological findings in the retinal pigment epithelium. Naturally, diseases of the macula are given particular attention, especially to age-related macular degeneration and the use of Anti-VEGF therapy. The wide spectrum of macular disorders has been expanded with attention given to retinal vascular disease, inflammatory, retinal and choroidal diseases, disorders of the optic nerve, and the typical findings of intraocular tumors, including choroidal melanomas, choroidal metastases and choroidal hemangiomas. The atlas »fluorescence angiography in Ophthalmology« by Dithmar and Holz provides an excellent perspective of the ophthalmic disorders that are relevant to the practice of clinical ophthalmology. It covers in graphic detail the pathological characteristics of macular, retinal, and choroidal diseases, and explains the findings that are necessary for the diagnosis, differential diagnosis and clinical management of ophthalmic diseases. With this, the atlas is a valuable resource for physicians, when used for teaching or in clinical practice, covering the elements necessary for proper diagnosis and management of ocular diseases. These are good reasons to praise the authors for their work and to expect that it will be enthusiastically received and widely adopted.

Heidelberg, October 2007

Prof. Dr. Hans E. Völcker
Chair of the Department of Ophthalmology
University of Heidelberg

Foreword

The development of imaging technologies for diagnostic application in clinical ophthalmology has made great strides forward in the past few years. With the further technical development of angiographic systems, the image quality in fluorescein and indocyanine green angiography has been considerably improved. In addition, a considerably more accurate method to study fundus autofluorescence is now available. The improvements in these diagnostic procedures has given us entirely new insights into the pathology of macular and retinal diseases, allowing us to better understand these disorders. This atlas is meant to provide a review of the fundamentals of fluorescein and indocyanine green angiography and also to offer numerous examples of the various distinguishing features and clinical signs of retinochoroidal diseases with practice-relevant case examples. With this in mind the selection of images has been given particular attention to quality (image resolution), and to the selection of clearly recognizable pathological features typical of the various diseases. The atlas provides a summarizing overview of the wealth and of diversity of the many angiographic findings found in patients with the various retinochoroidal diseases. It should also contribute to a more thorough knowledge of their differential diagnoses. Physicians not regularly engaged in the use of angiographic methods can also gain a better understanding of the various pathophysiological entities.

We would particularly like to express our appreciation to the engineers and physicists at Heidelberg Engineering, who have successfully brought the use of confocal scanning laser ophthalmoscopes in ophthalmic angiography to reality. We would also like to thank our colleagues at Springer publishing for their professional and efficient work in quickly preparing the book, given the rapidly advancing and expanding field of retinal imaging.

Heidelberg, Bonn, 2007

Stefan Dithmar
Frank G. Holz

Table of Contents

The physical and chemical fundamentals of fluorescence angiography

1.1   Fluorescence

Certain chemicals can be excited by electromagnetic radiation, i.e. they can absorb the radiant energy. Absorption of the radiant energy causes free electrons in such chemicals to be driven to higher levels of energy. These higher levels of energy are unstable, and the electrons fall back to their lower (pre-excitation) levels, and in so doing they emit the absorbed energy. This happens through the re-emission of electromagnetic radiation. The re-emitted radiation has less energy than the previously absorbed energy. Since the wavelength of electromagnetic radiation is inversely related to its energy content, the re-emitted energy always has a longer wavelength than the previously absorbed radiant energy. The energy so emitted is called **fluorescence**. The wavelengths of fluorescent light emitted by a particular chemical substance lie within a characteristic range called the **emission spectrum**.

Depending on the chemical to be excited, the electromagnetic energy (**excitation light**) must lie within a particular range of wavelengths called the **absorption spectrum**. Otherwise, the free electrons cannot be driven to higher levels of energy.

Fluorescence stops immediately when the excitation light is turned off, i.e. the emission occurs immediately after the absorption.

If the energy is emitted after a significant delay from the time of absorption, one speaks not of fluorescence, but phosphorescence.

1.2   Fluorescein

Fluorescein is a crystalline substance that is very water soluble (◘ Fig. 1.1). Its absorption spectrum lies between 465 and 490 nanometers, the blue light region of the shortest wavelengths in the visible spectrum. Its emission spectrum lies between 520 and 530 nanometers, meaning that fluorescein has a yellow-green fluorescence. The intensity of the fluorescence is pH dependent and reaches a maximum at the neutral pH of the blood. Even when greatly diluted, the fluorescence of the dye is easily detectable.

For fluorescence angiography of the ocular fundus, a 5 ml bolus of a 10% solution of sodium fluorescein is administered intravenously. With modern angiographic instruments (see below) the necessary quantity of dye can be significantly reduced.

Following the injection, 70 to 80% of the dye binds to plasma proteins. The remaining portion of fluorescein remains unbound and can diffuse through all vessel walls with the exception of the larger choroidal vessels, the retinal vessels (the inner blood-retinal barrier) and the cerebral vessels. The retinal pigment epithelium also forms a barrier to diffusion of the dye, since the RPE cells are bound to one another by tight junctions (zonulae occludentes) that form the outer blood-retinal barrier).

Due to the free passage of the unbound dye through vessel walls, skin and mucosal surfaces can acquire a yellowish tinge, most noticeably in the conjunctiva. The discoloration appears just a few minutes after the injection and can last for several hours. Fluorescein is eliminated through the liver and the kidneys, staining the urine a dark yellow-brown color. The dye is completely eliminated within 24 hours, provided that there is no impairment of renal function.

In some cases the injection of fluorescein can cause nausea, vomiting and dizziness, typically at about 5 minutes after the injection. These symptoms usually remit quickly. More serious

◘ **Abb. 1.1.** Fluorescein

reactions, such as anaphylactic shock, have been reported in small numbers of cases. Prior reports have estimated the incidence to be about 1 in 222,000 cases. More recent improvements in angiographic technique have reduced the necessary dose of fluorescein rather significantly and may have reduced the incidence even further. Never the less, it is vitally important that angiographic facilities always have appropriate drugs and personnel available for emergent use.

Contraindications for the intravenous use of fluorescein include: pregnancy, a history of prior severe reactions to fluorescein, and/or a history of severe allergic reactions in other settings.

1.3 Indocyanine Green

Indocyanine Green (ICG) is a tricarboxycyanine dye whose absorption spectrum and emission spectrum both lie within the infrared (absorption spectrum: 790 to 805 nanometers, emission spectrum: 825 to 835 nanometers) ($\blacksquare$ Fig. 1.2). Infrared radiation has a higher transmission than does visible light, and it can better penetrate tissues containing pigment (the melanin granules of the pigment epithelium), hemorrhages, or areas of exudation. 98% of intravascular ICG is bound to plasma proteins, a greater extent than that for fluorescein. In contradistinction to fluorescein, ICG is confined almost completely to the intravascular space. The fluorescent in-

tensity of ICG is weaker than that of fluorescein. For ICG angiography up to 25 mg of the dye is administered intravenously, while in fluorescein angiography (using modern angiographic systems) the necessary dose of fluorescein can be kept significantly lower. ICG is catabolized in the liver. It is in general well tolerated, and side effects are experienced less often than with injections of fluorescein. In the older literature the incidence of mortality following ICG injections is estimated to have been 1 in 333 thousand. ICG for injection is available as a solution that also contains 5% iodine as a stabilizer. This is in an inorganic form and its risks when used in patients with allergies to organic iodine are not known. For cases in which patients are known to have allergies to iodine and an ICG study is clinically indicated, instead of ICG one can use an iodine-free dye called infracyanine green. ICG angiography should not be used for patients with hyperthyroidism, allergies to shellfish, or poor liver function. ICG cannot cross the placental membrane, but there are no case studies in which it has been used during pregnancy.

ICG angiography is particularly well suited to the angiographic study of the choroidal circulation, since the infrared radiant energy has a higher transmission through the pigment epithelium than does the fluorescence emitted by fluorescein, and ICG in contradistinction to fluorescein does not pass through the vessel walls of the choriocapillaris.

$\blacksquare$ **Abb. 1.2.** Indocyanine Green

The Technical Fundamentals of Fluorescence Angiography

Present day methods of imaging fluorescein-angiograms, ICG-angiograms, and fundus auto-fluorescence use modified fundus cameras and scanning laser ophthalmoscopes (SLO). The development of scanning laser angiography has significantly improved the usefulness of fluorescence angiography. This chapter covers the fundamentals of scanning laser angiography.

2.1   The basic design of a scanning laser ophthalmoscope

■ Fig. 2.1 is a schematic diagram of the optical components of a scanning laser ophthalmoscope. Light from the laser source enters the scanner by passing through a beam splitter (BSP). The scanner itself consists primarily of 2 synchronized, oscillating mirrors that deflect the path of light in 2 dimensions. These impart a rapidly repetitive horizontal sweep (X axis) that is punctuated by incremental, vertical displacements of the horizontal sweeps (Y-axis) to form a series of individual, adjacent scanning lines (■ Fig. 2.2). In addition to the horizontal sweeps, the focal point of the laser beam can be axially deflected, meaning that the focal plane in the object being scanned can be shifted so as to produce a series of cross-sectional images that form a three dimensional optical reconstruction of the object being scanned. In addition to the oscillating mirrors, a telescope is also needed. By precise shifts

in the axial position of a lens in the telescope and varying the divergence or convergence of the light beam the focal plane of the scanner can be shifted in the axial dimension. Fluorescein molecules that are located in the focal place can absorb the photons, driving their free electrons to higher levels of energy content. On returning to their more stable, lower levels of energy content, the electrons release the energy, emitting photons that are red-shifted, i.e. are longer in wavelength and lower in energy content than the initially absorbed photons. The fluorescent light so emitted that manages to escape the eye

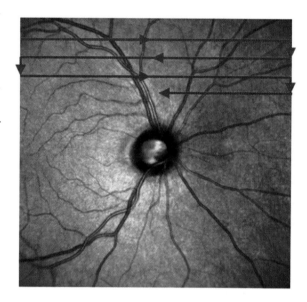

■ **Fig. 2.2.** Sampling pattern during image capture

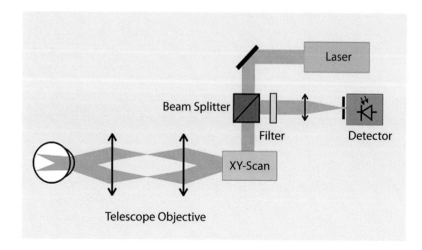

■ **Fig. 2.1.** Schematic structure of a confocal scanning laser ophthalmoscope

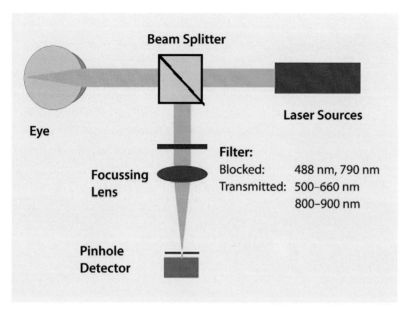

Eye

Beam Splitter

Laser Sources

Focussing Lens

Filter:
Blocked: 488 nm, 790 nm
Transmitted: 500–660 nm
                      800–900 nm

Pinhole Detector

Fig. 2.3. Schematic diagram of fluorescence detection

through the exit pupil is diverted by the beam splitter (BSP), directing the light into the path of a detector. To ensure that no light emitted by the laser will falsely elevate the measure, a filter is used to efficiently block the passage of the exciting light, while simultaneously allowing maximal transmission for the wavelengths of the emitted fluorescent light. The collimated beam of fluorescent light is made to converge on a small pinhole aperture (diameter circa 100 μm – **Fig. 2.3**), so that fluorescent light that originates in layers of tissue outside of the focal plane of the object, i.e. the retina, will be excluded from the image. This so-called confocal imaging permits a very efficient means of excluding stray light, which is especially useful when examining patients with cataractous lenses. This method significantly improves the contrast of the angiographic images.

2.2   Light Sources

In conventional fundus cameras bright flash lamps are used to flood the entire fundus with light, so that the entire frame of film or CCD chip is illuminated by the reflected light for several milliseconds. By contrast, the scanning laser ophthalmoscope images each pixel in serial fash-

ion, one after another. The typical illumination time per pixel is measured in nanoseconds and is therefore about one millionth of the time used for flash illumination. Due to the very short illumination time, the exciting light beam must be focused precisely on each successive pixel of the scanned object, for which purpose one needs a light source with a high degree spatial coherence. This has logically led to the adoption of scanning laser ophthalmoscopes as light sources for angiography

2.2.1   Lasers for Fluorescein Angiography

The most commonly administered ophthalmic contrast material for angiographic studies is fluorescein. It has an absorption maximum at circa 490 nm. The argon ion laser has been chosen for retinal fluorescein angiography, as in the Heidelberg Retina Angiograph (HRA, Heidelberg Engineering), since this laser has among its emitted wavelengths a strong emission line at 488 nm (**Fig. 2.4**). Gas lasers like the argon ion laser have several advantages, such as a low noise level and a favorable radiant profile. But they also have numerous disadvantages that make them rela-

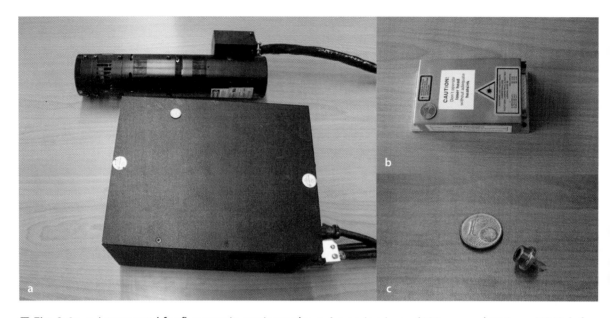

◘ Fig. 2.4a–c. Lasers used for fluorescein angiography: **a** Argon ion Laser (488 nm und 514 nm, HRA), **b** frequency doubling semiconductor laser (488 nm, HRA2), **c** Semiconductor laser diodes in the red or infrared spectral regions (e.g. ICG-Laser in HRA und HRA2)

tively expensive and unwieldy: operation of the laser cylinder requires costly power supplies that must both ignite the gas discharge and maintain the plasma flow with high levels of electrical current. In addition, the argon laser is relatively inefficient, requiring power input at kilowatt levels to generate laser output power at milliwatt levels. This means that the laser and its power supply must be ventilated with large volumes of cooling air. The average life span of the argon laser cylinder is about 5 years, and a gradual degradation of radiant output frequently requires replacement even before that. A suitable alternative to the argon laser with emissions of appropriate wavelengths has become commercially available just since 2002. The radiation of an optically pumped, semiconductor laser with strong infrared emissions at 976 nm is frequency doubled to a wavelength of 488 nm by means of a nonlinear crystal, and light of the primary wavelength is filtered out (◘ Fig. 2.4). To produce a comparable or better radiant stability, as compared to the argon ion laser, an expensive device for thermal regulation of the laser resonator is necessary. This is managed by a

multi-stage, thermoelectric, cooler coupled with a small fan to carry the heat out of the enclosure. The total electrical power consumption is modest, about 50 watts.

2.2.2 Lasers for red-free fundus imaging

In conjunction with angiographic studies a scanning laser ophthalmoscope can be used to capture red-free images of the fundus, i.e. fundus pictures taken with scanning lasers producing light in the blue or green regions of the spectrum. These are of particular interest, since many pathological structures, such as microaneurysms, have a very low contrast appearance when viewed with light of longer wavelengths and are difficult to see. In addition the nerve fiber bundles of the inner retina have a particularly high level of reflectance in the shorter wavelength regions of the spectrum (the »red-free« mode), improving the detection of localized defects which contrast more readily vis-à-vis adjacent areas of the fundus. The integrated semiconductor laser in the Heidelberg Retina Angiograph 2 (HRA 2, Heidelberg Engineering) used for fluorescein angiography (see above) can also be used for red-free photography. For this one need only remove the barrier filter which would otherwise absorb the light at 488 nm.

2.2.3 Lasers for Indocyanine green (ICG) angiography

Indocyanine green is excited by radiant energy in the infrared spectral region with an absorption maximum at 800 nm. In this spectral region simple diode lasers are available, such as those used in the entertainment industry. None the less care must be taken when choosing the spectral wavelengths for excitation of the dye, so as to ensure an optimal level of quality in the ICG-images. Given the large variation in the properties of available lasers, the angiographic laser diodes to be used must be specially selected and tested.

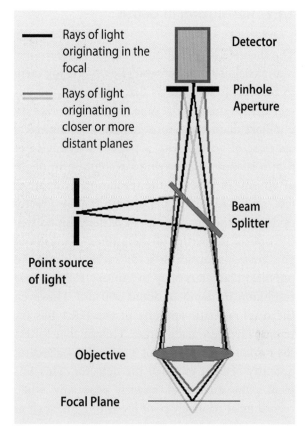

■ **Fig. 2.5.** The principle of confocal imaging

2.2.4 Lasers for reflective infrared imaging

Similarly, for the capture of infrared (IR) reflective images there are relatively simple IR laser diodes (wavelength region 810 to 830 nm) that can be used. The high variation in emitted wavelengths of lasers during commercial chip production is not as important as with ICG-angiography and a suitable device can be chosen without specific testing.

2.3 The Fundamentals of Optical Imaging

2.3.1 The confocal principle

■ Figure 2.5 is a schematic diagram of the principles of confocal imaging. A point source of light – a collimated laser beam is a point source of light along its entire pathway – is focused on the object plane by an optical imaging system. The returning (reflected or scattered) light is converged onto the aperture of a diaphragm that is positioned at a focal plane corresponding to the focal plane of the object. The diaphragm effectively suppresses light originating from nearer or farther planes of the three dimensional object being imaged. If the focal point is periodically shifted in a lateral direction (orthogonal to the optical axis) an image containing a two dimensional optical section of the object can be produced. If the focal plane is then periodically displaced deeper into the object, a series of equidistant parallel planes can be constructed, i.e. the object can be represented as a three dimensional volume. The HRA 2 enables the capture of such data sets that can be used, for example, to image the vascular bed of a tumor.

2.3.2 Resolution in depth

The theoretical resolution in depth, i.e. the minimum axial distance between two objects for them to be seen as separate, is determined by the numerical aperture of the objective, i.e. the ratio of pupillary diameter to focal length. The numerical aperture of an eye with a pupillary diameter of 6 mm is about 0.23, giving a resolution in depth of 80 μm. In practice, the resolution in depth is less, since wider pupillary apertures allow greater optical aberrations. Studies have determined that the optical properties of the human eye without any greater aberrations is diffraction limited at pupillary diameters of up to 3 mm, yielding a true resolution in depth of about 300 μm. However, the diaphragmatic aperture of the HRA has intentionally been made larger. This further lowers the resolution in depth, but it also allows a greater quantity of light to reach the detector. This improves the quality of images, especially when recording at relatively poor levels of light, such as those produced by autofluorescence or during the later phases of angiographic studies. Moreover, it is also desirable, especially during ICG angiography, to superimpose the fluorescent light arising from both the retinal and choroidal vessels in a combined image. This requires that the optical volume being portrayed in a two dimensional image combines signals from structures that are separated in depth by as much as 500 μm. The confocal aperture of the HRA2 is helpful in the suppression of stray light that originates in tissues other than the retina, such as the lens. This means that the confocal optics allow angiograms with good image resolution to be done in the eyes of patients with cataracts, which is not possible when using conventional image sensors like photographic film or CCD-chips. The products of peroxidation within the lens emit a fluorescence that results in a veil of gray light that covers the entire image, causing a substantial loss of contrast. In the images recorded by the HRA the contrast of structures in the retina is almost completely undiminished, since the confocal aperture completely blocks the fluorescence coming from the lens. Any impairment of the image quality is merely due to the unavoidable, low levels of laser light scattered by the cataract and by structures within the retina, thus reducing the strength of the fluorescence signal that reaches the detector.

2.3.3 Resolution in breadth

The resolution within a two dimensional image is determined by the size of the focal point (optical resolution). This in turn is theoretically dependent on the numerical aperture. In practice this diffraction limited resolution is, even in healthy eyes, attainable only up to a pupillary diameter of about 3 mm. In eyes with pupils more widely dilated than 3 mm the image quality is impaired by greater optical aberrations (astigmatism, coma and higher order aberrations) that are produced in the more peripheral portions of the lens. Despite the greater aperture and the greater quantity of light entering the eye, the image resolution at the retina is reduced. For this reason the HRA laser beam that strikes the pupil has been intentionally limited to a circle of 3 mm. The attainable resolution in an ideal eye can be calculated by the formula for Fraunhofer's diffraction. At a pupillary diameter of 3 mm this amounts to about 5 μm for light at 488 nm and about 8 μm for light at 800 nm. The digital sampling rate (pixel density) must be appropriate for this level of optical resolution. A higher sampling rate would not produce any improvement in the optical resolution.

2.4 The Heidelberg Retina Angiograph 2

The fluorescein angiography, Indocyanine green angiography and autofluorescence images, as well as the »red-free« and infrared images presented in this book were all captured by the Heidelberg Retina Angiograph 2 (HRA2), a product of Heidelberg Engineering GmbH, Heidelberg, Germany (❑ Fig. 2.6). As described above, theHRA2 is a confocal laser ophthalmoscope that has been designed specifically for high contrast and high resolution angiography of the retina.

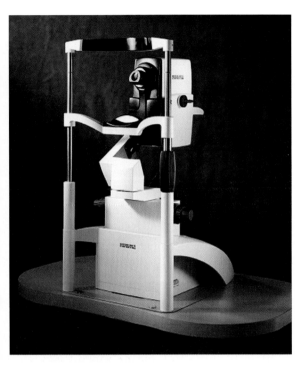

◘ Fig. 2.6. The Heidelberg Retina Angiograph 2 shown here with an instrument base equipped with an XYZ positioning control capability. Optionally, the HRA2 can also be mounted on an XY base

Standard autofluorescence images can be taken prior to administration of the dye when using the fluorescein angiography mode.

The parameters for these various operating modes are detailed in ◘ Table 2.1. One can chose to take single images, temporal sequences of images or depth sequences (so-called Z-scans) in any of the basic modes. The time based sequences are particularly important for studying the dynamics of vascular perfusion during the early phase of an angiogram. This is an important asset when searching for the locations of feeder vessels. Spherical refractive errors from -12 to +30 diopters can be compensated by setting the position of a control dial. In addition the examiner can select an internal myopic lens of -6 or -12 diopters, extending the total range of spherical correction (-24 to +30 diopters) without using any external lenses. Aside from the basic modes, the HRA2 provides other options that allow the examiner to maximize the useful range of the instrument, or alternatively to optimize the quality of the image. The most important characteristics are discussed in the following sections:

2.4.1 HRA2-Parameters for basic imaging modes

The HRA2 is used in the following basic modes:
- Fluorescein angiography (FA mode)   488 nm
- Indocyanine green angiography   790 nm
  (ICGA mode)
- Red-free reflection   488 nm
- Infrared reflection   820 nm

2.4.2 Simultaneous mode

In simultaneous mode synchronized pairs of images are taken with two laser sources sweeping in alternation. For example, simultaneous FA and ICGA images of identical areas can be captured and stored. This allows a direct and immediate comparison of the pathological findings in the two different angiographic modes. Similarly, si-

◘ Table 2.1

Field Size (Area)	HR: High Resolution Mode (Pixel Separation = 5 µm)		HS: High Refresh Mode (Pixel Separation = 10 µm)	
	Pixel Count	Refresh Rate	Pixel Count	Refresh Rate
30° x 30°	1536 x 1536	5 Hz	768 x 768	9 Hz
20° x 20°	1024 x 1024	7 Hz	512 x 512	13 Hz
15° x 15°	768 x 768	9 Hz	384 x 384	16 Hz

multaneous images can pair FA with IR reflection or red-free reflection with IR reflection

2.4.3 Composite mode

In addition to images of temporal series and depth sequences, so-called composite images can be captured. For this the operator pans the camera vertically and/or horizontally during the capture of single images. The software of the HRA2 automatically evaluates the images and connects them to one another, creating a large composite image (e.g. 100° by 80°). As part of this process the very rapid image analysis routines recognize any instances of eye movements during the capture sequence and compensate accordingly.

2.4.4 Fixation assistance

To ensure the patient's visual fixation is stable there are both internal and external fixation lights. The external light is mounted on a flexible arm and is freely moveable. The internal fixation device is an optional 3 by 3 matrix of LED's. In addition to a central fixation light there are 8 additional lights that can be used to examine peripheral retinal areas when necessary.

2.4.5 Wide angle objective

The standard objective is held in place by a simple bayonet coupling and can be easily removed to be replaced by a wide angle objective. With this special objective the width of field is broadened to 57°, which is particularly useful for the examination of structures in the peripheral fundus. The wide angle objective is automatically recognized by the camera and all of the basic modes (with some restrictions when capturing »red-free« reflective images) are available with the same sampling and refresh rate parameters at 57°, 35° and 27°. The wide angle objective can also be used in the composite mode, allowing even larger montage images of the fundus to be assembled.

2.4.6 ART module

The ART (automatic real time) module is a software application that detects and corrects for eye movements. When active, this module detects any movement of the fundus image in real time, compensating for translational, rotational, and shearing movements by comparison of each captured image to a spatially averaged (summated) reference image. This »real time mean image« is displayed continuously on the monitor and can be sampled and stored at any time. This significantly improves images that have weak signal to noise ratios, while excluding any artifacts caused by eye movement. This is particularly helpful when imaging autofluorescence and the later stages of angiograms, but also when examining eyes with clouded optical media or high astigmatism. In addition to this »ART mean« mode there is an »ART composite« mode which detects horizontal and vertical movements of the camera and displays a composite montage on the monitor in real time. This allows the examiner to judge the image quality in real time and to improve the appearance, for example, by rescanning areas that have been poorly imaged due to inadequate levels of illumination.

2.4.7 Examination of the anterior segment

Without any additional or external lenses, the HRA2 can be used to examine the anterior segment and to perform iris angiography. For this purpose one needs only to set the optics control to about +40 diopters and adjust the distance between camera and eye to optimize the focus.

2.4.8 Stereoscopic imaging

For precise analysis of complex structures (e.g. determining the course of specific vessels within choroidal neovascular lesions) it is often helpful to examine three dimensional images. The HRA2 is capable of producing stereoscopic views that serve this purpose. These consist of two successive single images (e.g. ICG angiographs) of an identical location that has been imaged from two different points of view. This is accomplished by capturing the two images in sequence from 2 different camera locations. After capture of the first image, the camera is shifted to one side by a distance of about 1 to 2 mm, whereupon the second image is captured. When viewed binocularly, the image disparity evokes a stereoscopic impression. Looking at these stereo pairs with a special stereo viewer, the examiner can gain a very helpful, three dimensional impression of the scanned structures.

2.4.9 Components of the analytical software

The analysis software of the HRA2, in addition to the above mentioned components for stereoscopic imaging, the playing of temporal sequences or Z-scans and the computation of »mean« and composite images, includes other important functions: areas in stored images can be marked and labeled, and the images can then be converted to other image modes. Biometric functions for the measurement of linear distances, the sizes of marked areas, and their mean gray level values are also available to the examiner.

Normal Fluorescence Angiography and General Pathological Fluorescence Phenomena

3.1   Normal Fluorescence Angiography and general pathological fluorescence phenomena

The time from when an injection of fluorescein is administered into an antecubital vein until the time that the dye first appears in the central retinal artery is called the arm-retina-time and it can vary significantly (between circa 7 to 15 seconds). It depends on a number of factors, including the size of the cubital vein, the speed of the injection, the blood pressure and cardiac output. It is shorter in young people and longer in the elderly. The dye appears first in the choroid and then shortly thereafter in the central retinal artery. There is no standard nomenclature for the various phases. Generally, though, an early phase is identified as the time to filling of the retinal arterioles (arterial phase), an intermediate phase (»arteriovenous phase«) that lasts up to the first appearance of the dye in retinal veins (and often subdivided into early, intermediate and late arteriovenous phases), and finally a late phase during which the fluorescence gradually fades away. Late phase images are usually taken from 5 to 10 minutes after the injection, but in some cases it can be helpful to take even more images later on.

3.1.1   Choroid

In normal fluorescein angiographic studies the dye appears initially in the large choroidal vessels and then shortly later in the choriocapillaris (◘ Fig. 3.1). The choriocapillaris is made up of numerous lobules, each having a size that is about one fourth that of the optic disc (◘ Fig. 3.2). The lobules fill independently from one another, giving a transiently patched or blotched appearance (◘ Fig. 3.1b). This is to be distinguished from pathological filling defects in the choriocapillaris (◘ Fig. 3.2). The visibility of choroidal perfusion depends on the degree of pigmentation in the retinal pigment epithelium. The fenestrated capillaries of the choriocapillaris allow molecules of the dye to escape diffusely into the choroid, so that details of the choroidal circulation are no longer visible through the background fluorescence.

3.1.2   Cilioretinal vessels

Any cilioretinal vessels are fed by ciliary vessels and appear with the choroidal circulation. They are easily recognizable just before the delayed appearance of the dye in the retinal circulation (◘ Fig. 3.3).

3.1.3   Optic disc

The prelaminar portion of the optic nerve is fed primarily by the peripapillary choroidal vessels. Thus, the capillaries of the optic disc become visible in synchrony with the choroidal perfusion.

3.1.4   Retinal vessels

About 1 to 3 seconds after choroidal perfusion begins, fluorescence appears in the central retinal artery. Several factors make study of the retinal vascular bed particularly good: the blood supply arises at a single point, the retinal pigment epithelium (RPE) provides a nicely contrasting background, and the larger retinal vessels all remain in a single plane. The fluorescein flows at first into the central retinal circulation, with the consequence that its venous flow first appears in the larger veins. The venous flow in the central retinal circulation first appears in the larger veins in a typically laminar pattern (◘ Fig. 3.1). With this the early venous phase begins. A short while later the fluorescein fills the peripheral retinal veins, completing an angiographic image of the entire retinal venous bed.

3.1.5   Macula

In a fluorescein angiogram the central macular region appears darker than the surrounding retina, since the yellow macular pigment (Lutein and Zeaxanthin) absorbs some of the blue light needed to produce fluorescence. Furthermore, the macular RPE has a higher content of melanin than does the extramacular RPE, so that the exciting radiant energy and the emitted choroidal fluorescence are both partially blocked (❏ Fig. 3.1)

3.1.6 Sclera

The last tissue to fluoresce is the innermost layer of the sclera. The is particularly visible in areas where no RPE and no choriocapillaris cover the sclera (❏ Figs. 3.4 and 3.5).

3.1.7 Iris

With the assistance of fluorescein angiography, processes in the anterior segment can be revealed, such as iris lesions (e.g. tumors and/or vascular lesions) (❏ Fig. 3.6).

3.2 Normal ICG-Angiography

The early phase of an ICG angiogram is characterized by the appearance of the dye in the choroidal circulation, which is normally the case during the first minute following the injection. The large choroidal vessels and then also the large retinal vessels are easily visible. In the mid phase the choroidal veins are also seen, thought not quite as well, and a homogeneous choroidal hyperfluorescence appears. During the late phase, about 15 minutes after the injection, there are no longer any identifiable details in the choroidal or retinal circulation. The optic disc is dark and the choroidal vessels become hypofluorescent.

3.3 Pathological fluorescence phenomena

Specific angiographic pathological findings will be discussed with their associated disorders. Generally one can divide the pathological fluorescence

phenomena into hyper- and hypofluorescence. When interpreting fluorescence phenomena, the origin of the fluorescence and the temporal angiographic phase should be considered. During the course of the angiogram, hypo- and hyperfluorescence can alternate in the same locations. So a transition from an initial hypofluorescence to a later hyperfluorescence is typically seen in inflammatory disorders of the retina and choroid. It begins with a blockage of the background fluorescence, caused by retinal edema, and evolves later on into a hyperfluorescence caused by an inflammatory increase in vascular permeability.

3.3.1 Hyperfluorescence

Hyperfluorescence may be defined as a greater level of fluorescence than would be found in an otherwise normal angiogram. There are two fundamental causes of hyperfluorescence:

Window defect
The retinal pigment epithelium weakens the transmission of fluorescein fluorescence. A defect within the RPE allows an increased transmission of the normal choroidal fluorescence. At the location of the RPE defect a sharply defined area of hyperfluorescence appears that does not change in size or shape during the angiogram (a window defect). Also in the region of a central retinal defect (a macular hole) fluorescence is elevated, since the site of the defect has no luteal macular pigment, which would otherwise partially block transmission of choroidal fluorescence.

Increased accumulation of fluorescent dye
The term »**leakage**« refers to the escape of fluorescein from vessels with pathologically increased permeability. During angiography there is a progressive increase in the size and intensity of extra-vascular hyperfluorescence. By »**pooling**« we mean the accumulation of fluorescein in an anatomical space. An example of this is serous elevation of the RPE (▶ Chapter 5.1.5) in which the fluorescein from the choriocapillaris collects in the space- beneath the elevated pigment epi-

thelium. Another example is central serous retinopathy (► Chapter 5.7) in which pooling of the dye collects beneath a circumscribed region of retinal elevation. »**Staining**« refers to accumulation of fluorescein within a tissue. Staining is also seen in normal tissues (◘ Figs. 3.4 and 3.5) as well as in pathologically altered tissues, (e.g. disciform scars, ► Chapter 5.1.9).

3.3.2 Hypofluorescence

Hypofluorescence refers to a weakened level of fluorescence, when compared to normal angiographic studies. For hypofluorescence there are again two different basic disturbances at fault.

Blocking of fluorescence

Loss of media clarity, vitreous hemorrhages, subhyaloid hemorrhages and intraretinal bleeding can weaken or completely block fluorescent light (◘ Fig. 3.7). Subretinal pathological processes block choroidal fluorescence, while leaving retinal fluorescence undiminished.

Vascular filling defects

Reduced or elevated levels of tissue perfusion can likewise result in hypofluorescence. This is often seen in retinal vascular occlusions and also following interrupted blood flow in the papillary and peripapillary fundus. Choroidal vascular occlusions, on the contrary, are much more difficult to detect by fluorescein angiography.

◘ **Fig. 3.1a–f.** A patient with circumscribed retinal vascular anomalies superotemporal to the optic disc (left eye). **a** Fundus image. **b–f** Aside from the vascular anomalies, a normal fluorescein angiogram. **b** Initially mottled, delayed filling of the choroid. **c** Then a progressive filling of the retinal arterial vessels. **d** Laminar blood flow in the large retinal veins. **e** An arteriovenous phase with complete filling of all arteries and veins of the retinal circulation. **f** In the late phases a gradual fading of the fluorescence.

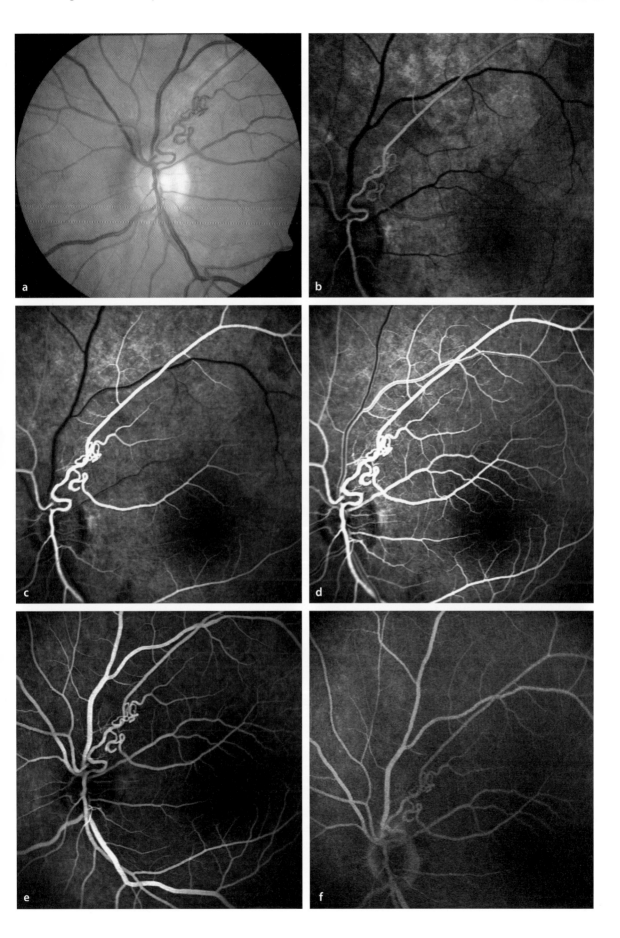

◘ **Fig. 3.2a–f.** A 20 year old patient with »patchy vision« in the right eye, 20/20 acuity, and myopia of -9 diopters. **a** Ophthalmoscopy shows a rather bright, myopic fundus appearance with no unusual features. **b–f** Fluorescein angiographic sequence. Due to the myopia there is reduced RPE pigmentation, making the choroidal circulation easily visible. In the early phase there is a distinct disturbance of perfusion in the choriocapillaris, particularly in the peripapillary fundus. Some lobules of the cho-riocapillaris appear to be unperfused. In the lower right corner, one can see a single lobule of the choriocapillaris with its feeding vessel. This is easily distinguished from the surrounding areas because neighboring lobules of the choriocapillaris are unperfused. With increasing departure of fluorescein from the choriocapillaris, there is a diffuse background fluorescence that obscures the choroidal vessels. **f** Filling of the entire retinal circulation is complete.

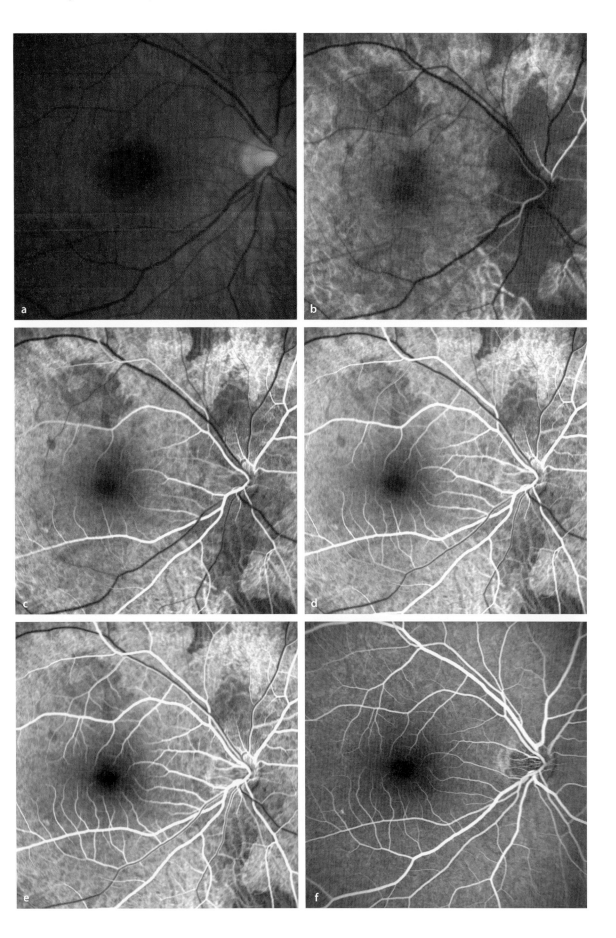

◘ Fig. 3.3a–f. Simultaneous fluorescein-/ICG-angiography. **a** Fluorescein angiogram. One can see uneven filling of the choriocapillaris lobules in the early phase. Simultaneous with the choroidal filling (and still prior to perfusion of the retinal circulation) a single cilioretinal vessel fills with dye. **b** The corresponding ICG angiogram shows choroidal and cilioretinal vessels. The image is brightly illuminated by the sudden appearance of choroidal hyperfluorescence. The retinal vessels have not yet filled, and appear as black lines. **c** Fluorescein angiography. In the next phase the retinal arterioles fill with dye. In addition laminar flow can now be seen in the inferotemporal vein. **d** The matching ICG-angiogram. The intensity of the ICG-choroidal fluorescence has already begun to diminish and the choroidal vessels are more easily distinguishable. **e, f** The arteriovenous phase with complete filling of the arterial and venous retinal vessels.

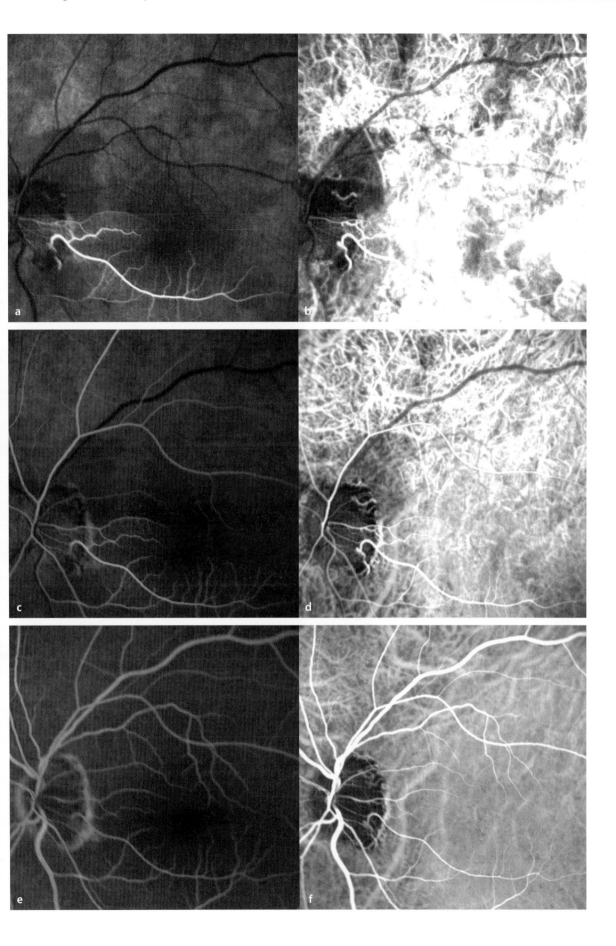

Fig. 3.4a–d. A 22 year old patient, right eye. Acuity 20/20. **a** A coincidental finding is a retinal-choroidal coloboma inferior to the disc. Through this defect one can see the dome-shaped, posteriorly evaginated, white scleral coat. A few choroidal vessels course over the inner sclera surface. The choriocapillaris is missing. Hyperplasia of the RPE can be seen on the edge of the coloboma. **b** Autofluorescence: Within the coloboma, complete extinction of autofluorescence. **c** Fluorescein angiography: Within the coloboma, dye fills the large choroidal vessels. Due to the absence of choriocapillaris, the coloboma appears hypofluorescent. **d** In the later course of the fluorescein angiogram one can see staining of the inner sclera surface, causing the coloboma to now appear hyperfluorescent.

Fig. 3.5a,b. A patient with high myopia, paracentral foci of chorioretinal ectasias, and peripapillary atrophy. Fluorescein angiography. **a** In the early phase filling defects in the region of the ectasias due to atrophy of the choriocapillaris. **b** In the last phase, one can see staining of the sclera as foci of hyperfluorescence.

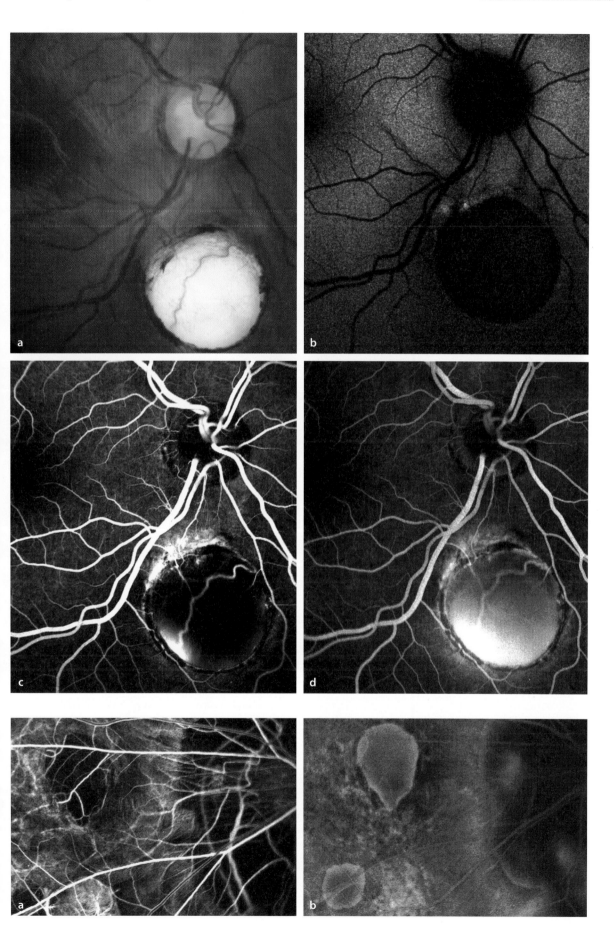

■ **Fig. 3.6a–d.** A 20 year old patient with congenital vascular anomalies of the iris. **a** Clinical appearance. **b–d** The fluorescein angiogram clearly shows the course of the affected vessels, and the normal vascular architecture of the iris is recognizable.

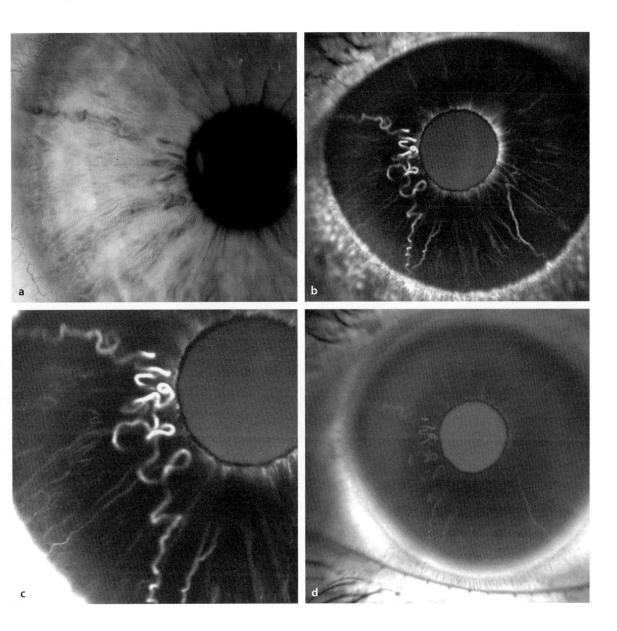

⬛ Fig. 3.7a–f. A 30 year old patient with vitreous clouding in the left eye, caused by uveitis. **a–f** Simultaneous fluorescein (**a, c, e**) and ICG (**b, d, f**) angiography. The vitreous cloud causes a shadowing of the fluorescence phenomenon. With fixation movement during angiography it can be easily seen that the shadowed area moves about, identifying its source as located in the vitreous body.

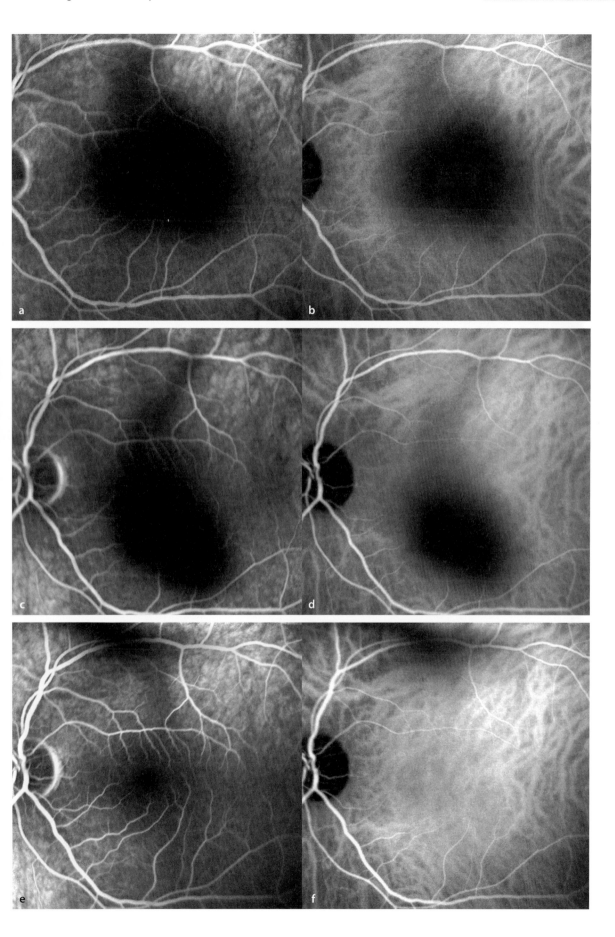

Fundus Autofluorescence

4.1   Introduction

Fundus autofluorescence (FAF) images can mark the effects of aging and disease at the level of the retinal pigment epithelium. The *in vivo* detection of FAF relies primarily on the presence of fluorophors in the lipofuscin (LF) granules of RPE cells, including the bis-retinoid pigment A2-E. With aging the post mitotic RPE cells accumulate LF granules in the cytoplasm, accompanied by a reduction in the density of the melanin granules. Excessive accumulation of LF (and its characteristic FAF signal) is a marker for multifactorial and degenerative maculopathies, including age related macular degeneration (AMD), idiopathic central serous chorioretinopathy, and purely inherited monogenetic diseases such as Best's vitelliform degeneration and Stargardt's disease. Until recently, accumulation of RPE lipofuscin could be determined only by fluorescence microscopy. Information about the specific LF content of the RPE and the topographical distribution of its intensity could not be determined by methods other than conventional imaging technologies, including fundus photography, fluorescence angiography or optical coherence tomography. FAF imaging provides another method that can help confirm the diagnosis, differentiate the phenotype, and recognize new prognostic factors, particularly when evaluating AMD. FAF now contributes to our understanding of the pathophysiological role of the RPE as a final common pathway for many retinal and macular diseases. Moreover, it helps with identification of the distribution and density of the macular pigments lutein and zeaxanthin.

4.2   Scanning laser ophthalmoscopy and modified fundus photography

In vivo images of optimal quality and resolution can be captured by confocal scanning laser ophthalmoscopy (cSLO) using the HRA classic, the HRA2 or the Spectralis HRA/OCT instrument (Heidelberg Engineering). Alternatively, there are modified fundus cameras available. A confocal system has the advantage that, with an additional diaphragm, light reflected from the plane of focus is selectively detected. Recent improvements in the design of the cSLO now allow a resolution of up to 5μm/pixel, which is sufficient to resolve images at the level of individual RPE cells.

4.3   Methods

4.3.1   Fundamentals

The cSLO, developed by many users, is an instrument that projects monochromatic light through a confocal optical system onto the ocular fundus and detects the reflected light returning from the corresponding focal plane The confocal property minimizes the stray light returning from outside the focal plane, which increases the image contrast. With this method the reflected light from individual retinal points can be properly ordered, producing a scanned, analog signal that is displayed on a monitor. The image can be stored and digitally processed. For the capture of fundus fluorescence, an exciting light with a wavelength of 488 nm is projected onto the fundus, and the image derived from emissions above 500 nm is captured. Optimal image quality requires the use of a barrier filter to block the short wavelength light used for excitation. The maximal light level (about 2 mW/cm2) lies well below the allowable limits set by international standards.

4.3.2   The operational sequence of a fundus examination with the cSLO

Prior to imaging fundus autofluorescence, the infrared mode of the camera is first used with the auxiliary lens in place to focus the fundus image. After switching to the »fluorescein angiography« mode the sensitivity of the camera is manually calibrated so that the retinal vessels and the optic disc are clearly visible. Care is taken to avoid excessive levels of light that would lead to an overexposure. Next, a series of 6 to 24 single autofluorescence images are recorded. Since FAF arising from LF is considerably weaker that the fluorescence of the angiographic dye fluorescein, a suitable fluorescence intensity is automatically determined by appropriate software (Heidelberg Eye Explorer) and chosen from among the series of images. By experience a mean of 6 to 10 individual images will allow determination of an optimal level of amplification of the FAF signal. Following injection of a fluorescent dye, appropriate images of FAF are no longer possible.

4.3.3 Lipofuscin in the retinal pigment epithelium

The RPE plays an essential role in the normal function of the neurosensory retina. In particular the permanent phagocytosis and lysosomal catabolism of photoreceptor outer segments (POS) by post mitotic RPE cells is essential for normal photoreceptor function. With advancing age there is a gradually increasing failure of the breakdown of photoreceptor discs, leading to an accumulation of LF in the lysosomal compartment of RPE cells. Retinal disorders, such as Best's disease, Stargardt's disease or retinitis pigmentosa accelerate the accumulation of excessive LF, causing vision problems to appear in younger patients. There are numerous experimental and clinical indications that excessive accumulation of LF above some critical level can lead to loss of function and eventual cell death. The LF granules contain toxic molecular components, such as A2 E, that interfere with several molecular mechanisms that are necessary for the normal function of the RPE cells. Clinical studies have shown that regions of elevated FAF are associated with loss of retinal sensitivity and these regions coincide with the geographic atrophy that marks the development and spread of the degeneration.

4.3.4 Normal fundus autofluorescence

The normal FAF image is characterized by low levels of fluorescence in the optic disc (absence of LF), along the retinal blood vessels (blockage of fluorescence by the blood columns lying anterior to the RPE cells), and a central zone of reduced fluorescence intensity caused by absorption by the yellow pigments of the macula (lutein and zeaxanthin). Not only LF granules possess the fluorophors that emit the autofluorescence recorded by these imaging techniques. Fluorophors can be found in practically all tissues, although with varying spectral properties and intensities of the light emitted. Thus, fluorophors are present in the choroid and the sclera. In the absence of RPE cells the large choroidal vessels are recognizable in the autofluorescence mode, since the vascular walls are autofluorescent. In normal studies these signals play no role, since the blue excitation light is largely absorbed by the intact layer of RPE cells. The quality of FAF images depends in part on the clarity of the media. Cataracts in particular are associated with an absorption phenomenon, due to their dark yellow brunescence that absorbs the blue laser light. Similarly, corneal and vitreal clouding are also associated with impairment of FAF image quality. For these reasons quantification of the autofluorescence level at specific retinal locations by the monochromatic method would not be ideal; instead, the use of topographic image data (i.e. the registration of FAF patterns) is more readily useful.

4.4 Fundus autofluorescence – typical findings

Changes in the topographic distribution of FAF intensity are found in a number of retinal diseases that often show characteristic patterns.

In Stargardt's disease, for example, one typically finds a normal funduscopic appearance, while the FAF images have areas of heightened fluorescence (due to LF accumulation) or depressed fluorescence (where the RPE is atrophic).

Best's disease manifests as diffusely elevated levels of FAF with an additional increase of fluorescence intensity in the area of the funduscopically visible yellow deposit that characterizes the vitelliform lesion. This is also the case for pattern dystrophies, including adult vitelliform macular dystrophy.

FAF findings in cases of retinitis pigmentosa and other photoreceptor dystrophies reflect secondary changes appearing at the level of the retinal pigment epithelium. In some types one can also find an accumulation of LF granules in the pigment epithelium, and areas of atrophy are precisely defined. Frequently one finds a ring of increased autofluorescence at 4–5° of eccentricity from the fovea, the so-called »rod-ring« (Fig. 4.10).

Eyes with AMD show a wide spectrum of FAF changes in association with the various stages of disease. In early cases of AMD, there are areas of elevated FAF. These areas don't correspond to visible findings like retinal drusen, however, and they are highly variable. Focal areas of hyperpigmentation are almost always accompanied by elevated FAF (melanolipofuscin); areas of retinal drusen are heterogeneous, and can have elevated, reduced or normal levels of FAF.

Areas of geographic atrophy in the advanced stages of AMD are characterized by a marked reduction in FAF, since in these areas the RPE and its autofluorescent lipofuscin have been destroyed. At the margins of these atrophic areas one finds a variety of FAF patterns. Atrophic areas with diffusely elevated FAF at their margins advance more rapidly than atrophic areas with no or only focally elevated FAF. Phenotypic categorization, based on the FAF appearance, allows a prognostic determination of non-exudative AMD in its later stages. In contradistinction to the drusen of AMD, hereditary drusen, which arise at an earlier age, have a generally higher level of autofluorescence (Fig. 4.1d). This finding suggests that hereditary drusen have different molecular structures or higher densities of LF granules in the overlying RPE, than do the drusen of AMD. Similarly, pigment epithelial detachments (PED) produce a heterogeneous FAF signal; this, however, seems to be determined more by the stage of the PED itself, rather that the underlying disease process. Elevated FAF intensity could also arise from the fluorophors in the extracellular fluid between the RPE and Bruch's membrane. Drusen of the optic nerve head are to be differentiated from the drusen of AMD or those of hereditary retinal diseases. Here, the elevated FAF has to do with the calcification of degenerated axonal remnants. A prominently elevated FAF of the optic disc is useful in the differential diagnosis of optic disc elevations of uncertain origin (Fig. 8.3). Keep in mind when evaluating FAF fundus images that other structures – in addition to the RPE-LF – can be autofluorescent, e.g. old blood products.

Fig. 4.1a–d. In images of the mono-layer of polygonal cells in the RPE : **a** one finds the lipofuscin granules are most densely packed closer to the cell membrane. In the schematic diagram **b** is the typical distribution of lipofuscin (yellow) and melanin (brown) granules. The cell nucleus is found in the basal cytoplasm, while the melanin granules are more densely packed in the central apical zone. **c** In FAF images of the normal RPE one finds low levels of fluorescence marking the paths of retinal blood vessels, since their blood columns are located anterior to the RPE (the blockage phenomenon). In the central macular region is a reduced level of FAF caused by absorption of the fluorescence by the macular pigments (lutein and zeaxanthin). **d** With appropriate image processing software, several adjacent images can be merged into a composite montage. One can see the locations of hereditary drusen. Their points of elevated fluorescence are most densely located in the macula, but are also scattered through retinal areas that are far outside of the macular region.

4.4 · Fundus autofluorescence – typical findings

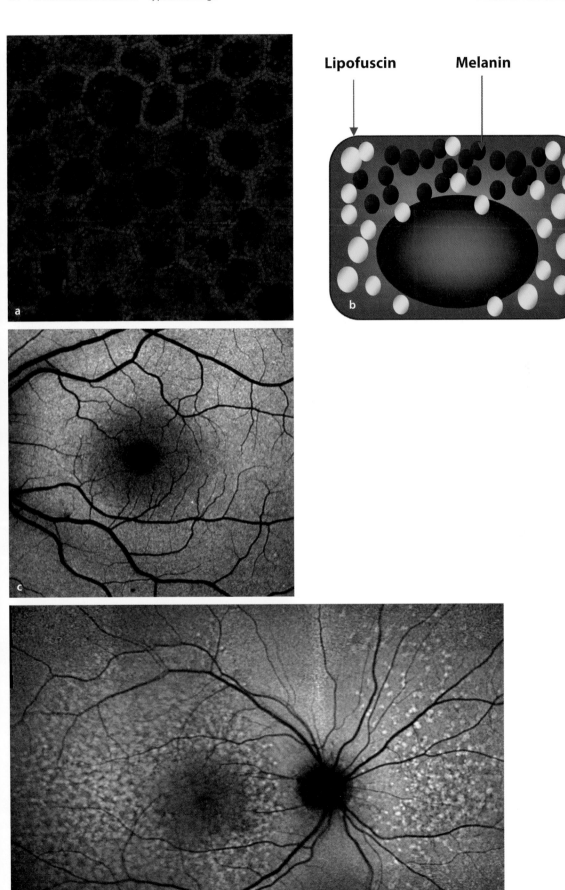

Lipofuscin   Melanin

▣ Fig. 4.2a–c. Geographic atrophy, seen here in a case of AMD, is characterized by a strong reduction in FAF, caused by an absence of vital RPE cells and their fluorescent lipofuscin. By contrast, as seen here, the borders of this atrophic area have an elevated level of fluorescence **a** (colored areas in 3D image). Over a 5 year period, one can see that expansion of the atrophic area in this 67 year old patient occurred at the margins of the lesion where excessive accumulation of LF had previously been located **b, c.**

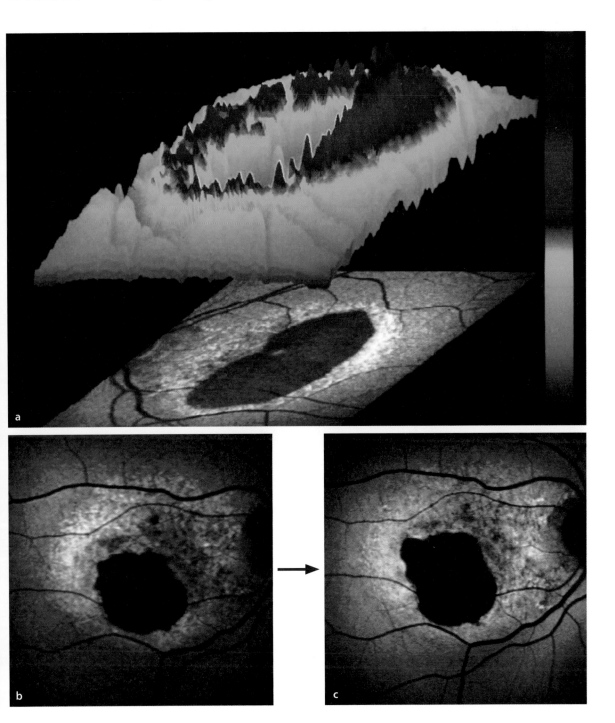

■ Fig. 4.3a–f. Three examples of fundus autofluorescence in the presence of the geographic atrophy of AMD. The atrophy itself shows a corresponding, strong reduction of the FAF signal as a consequence of absent vital RPE cells. One can see patterns of abnormally elevated autofluorescence in the margins of these lesions. While the example in **a** and **b** at the top shows a ribbon of elevated FAF signal at the margin, the two other examples below have a more diffusely distributed pattern of FAF outside the atrophic areas. Note that the variable FAF levels outside the atrophic areas are not accompanied by any visible changes in the fundus photographs.

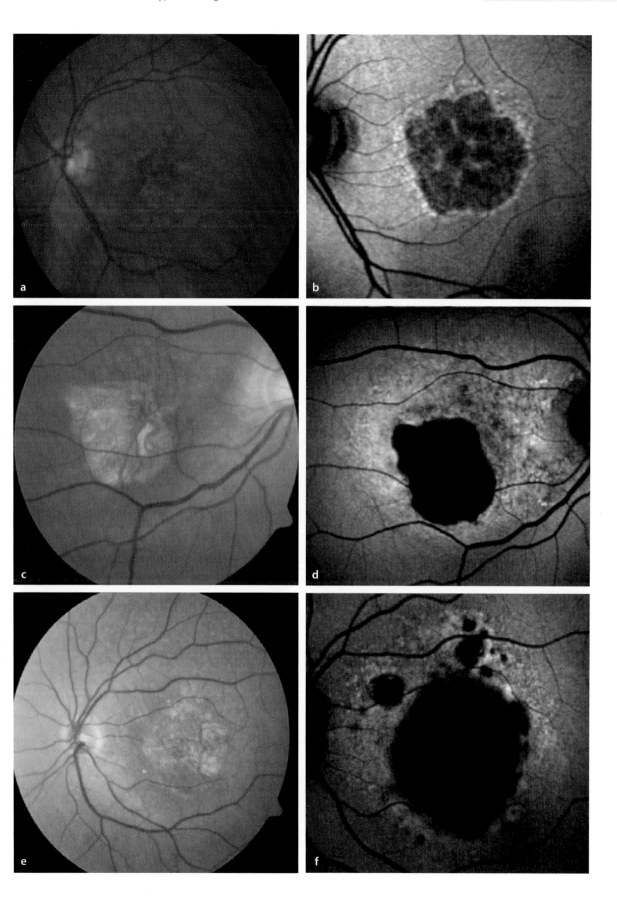

■ **Fig. 4.4a–f.** Three additional examples of FAF images in three different patients with the geographic atrophy of AMD. One can see a pronounced intra- individual left/right symmetry and marked inter-individual variability in the appearance of the atrophic areas and their margins of elevated FAF.

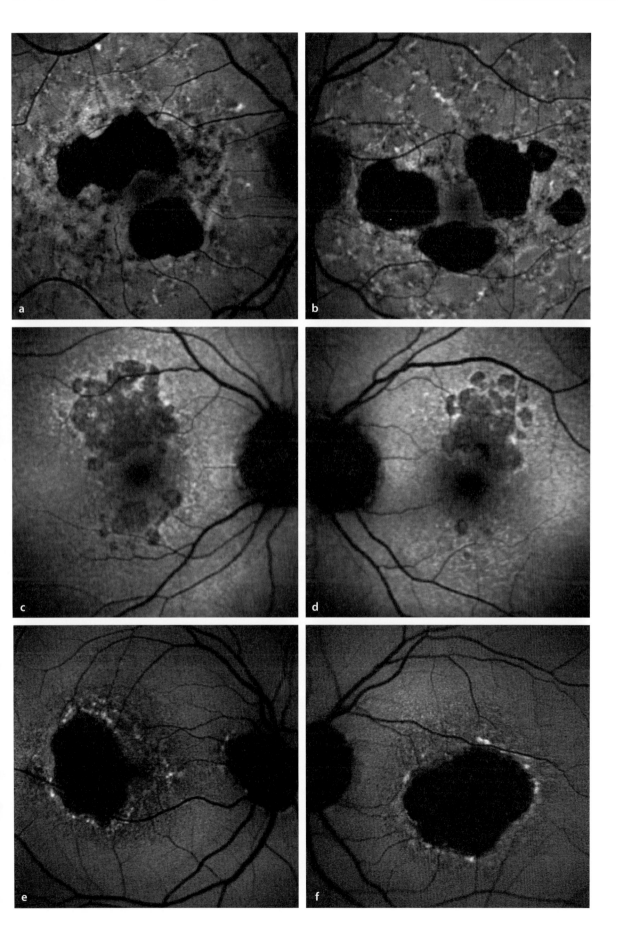

Fig. 4.5a–f. Examples of reticulated drusen both without **a, b** and with **c–f** associated geographic atrophy. Reticulated drusen can be easily identified in FAF images. They can be accompanied by both hyper- and hypo-intense areas of autofluorescence.

4

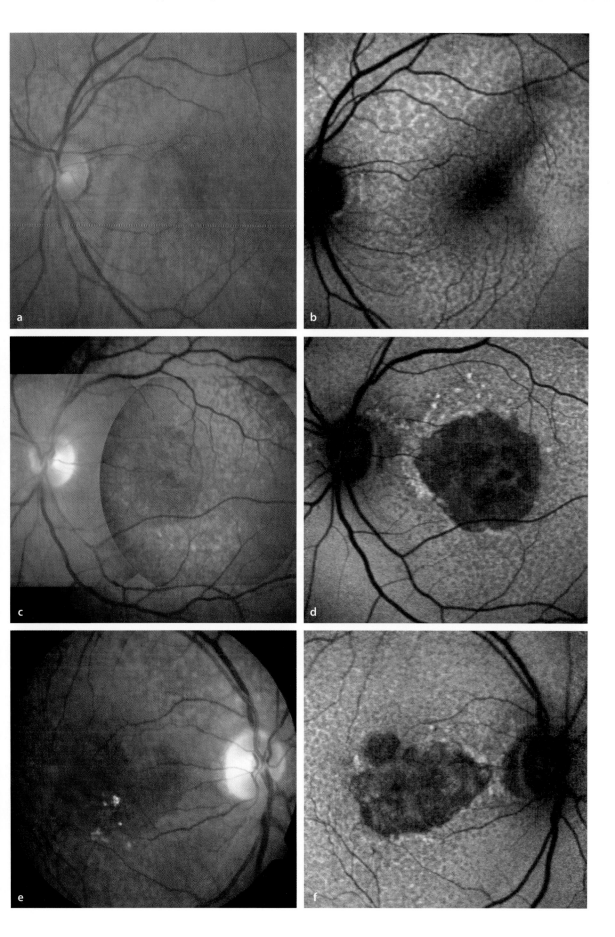

Fig. 4.6a–f. In cases of fundus flavimaculatus, or Stargardt's disease, there are characteristic yellow flecks at the level of the RPE with increased autofluorescence due to an excess accumulation of lipofuscin **a–d.** The lowest pair of images **e, f** are from a case of late onset Stargardt's disease with a confirmed ABCA4-mutation (67 years old; first symptoms after the age of 50). There is a central zone of atrophy with a corresponding central area of diminished autofluorescence, due to an absence of RPE cells. The appearance mimics the geographic atrophy of age-related macular degeneration, but a clear distinction can be made by the peripheral presence of typical yellow flecks with elongated (pisciform) shapes.

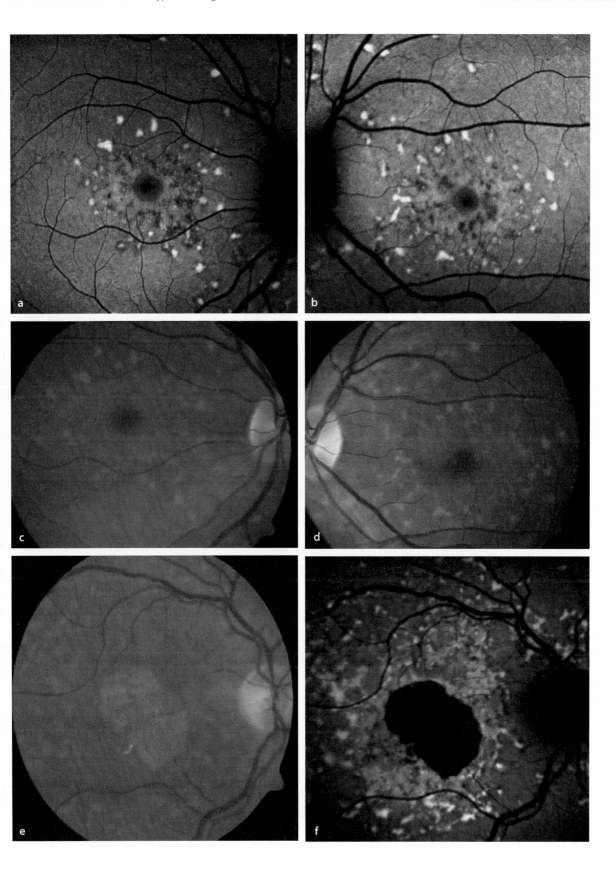

◨ Fig. 4.7. Classification of the fundus autofluorescence changes outside the central area of geographic atrophy, using terminology recently introduced in the literature*. The different phenotypes also have prognostic relevance, i.e. progression of the central atrophic areas is related to the patterns of abnormal fluorescence. In eyes with no elevated autofluorescence at the margins of the atrophic zone ('none') there is only a very slow increase in size, while the 'trickling' pattern is associated with a very high rate of progression. This is also relevant for interventional studies when recruiting subjects with the highest likelihood of rapid progression.

*A Bindewald, S Schmitz-Valckenberg, JJ Jorzik, J Dolar-Szczasny, H Sieber, C Keilhauer, A Weinberger, S Dithmar, D Pauleikhoff, U Mansmann, S Wolf, FG Holz for the FAM Study Group. Classification of abnormal fundus autofluorescence patterns in the junctional zone of geographic atrophy in patients with AMD. *Br J Ophthalmol* 2005;89:874–878

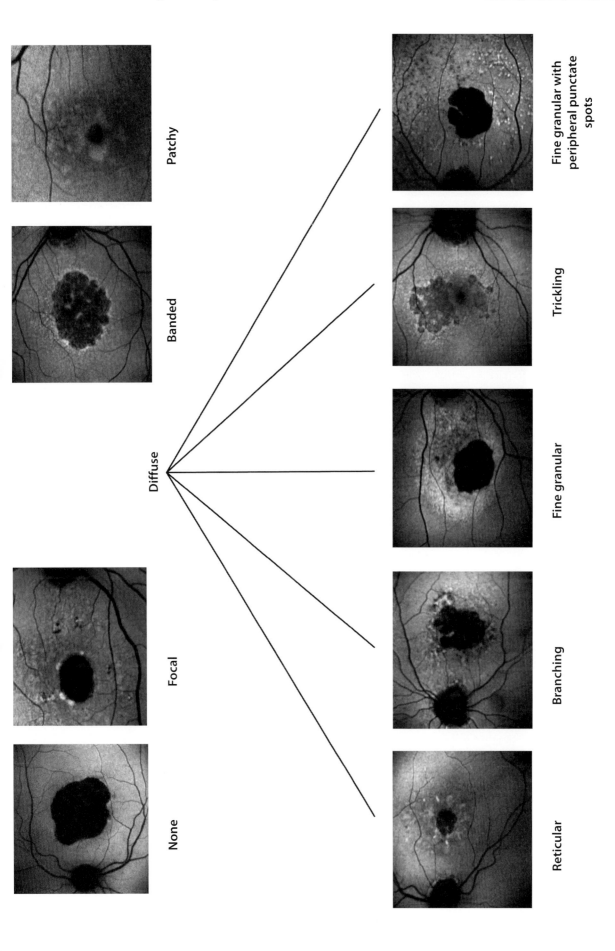

Patchy

Banded

Diffuse

Focal

None

Fine granular with peripheral punctate spots

Trickling

Fine granular

Branching

Reticular

◨ **Fig. 4.8a–f.** A 55 year old patient with multifocal Best's disease. The yellow (vitelliform) lesions **a,b** have a strongly elevated signal intensity due to increased levels of stored lipofuscin **c,d**. While these lesions are only partially hypofluorescent in fluorescein angiograms, they appear black during Indocyanine-green angiography **f**. Apparently the yellow vitelliform material absorbs much of the laser's infrared light.

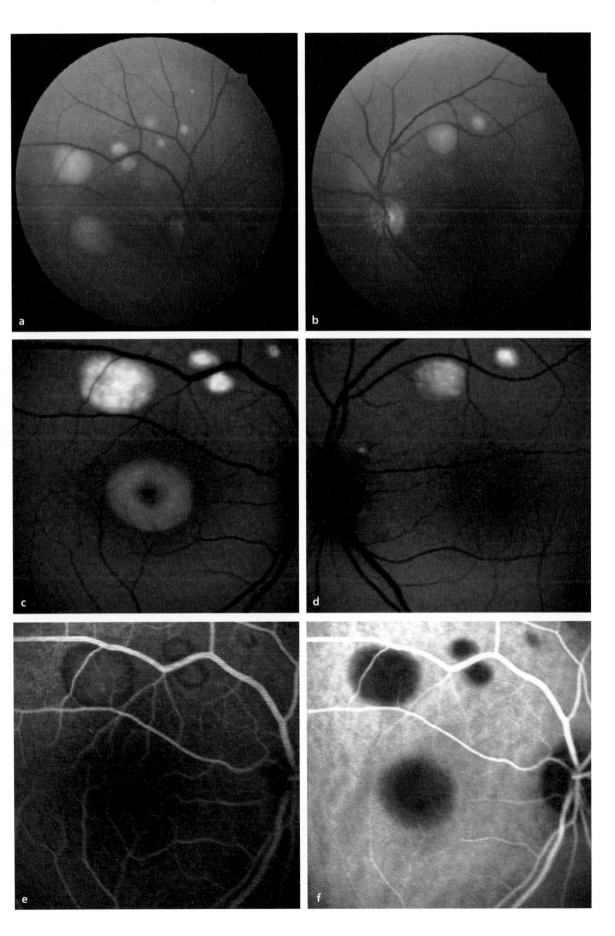

◼ **Fig. 4.9a–d.** A 27 year old patient with autosomal recessive macular dystrophy (Kjellin's disease). The yellow flecks in the posterior pole **a,b** have a central zone of elevated autofluorescence and a surrounding halo of reduced autofluorescence **c,d**. Halos like these would be very atypical for drusen. The morphological correlates for this phenomenon in Kjellin's disease are unknown. These fundus findings are accompanied by functional neurological deficits, including spastic paraplegia, mental retardation and muscular atrophy.

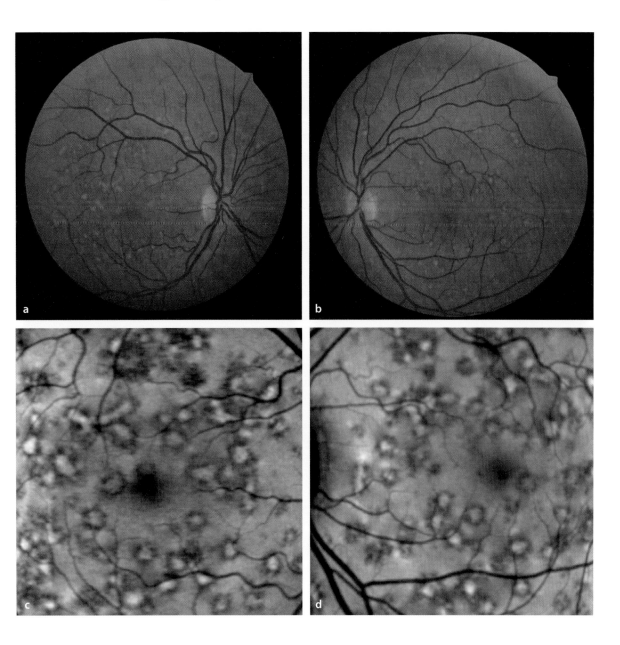

◨ **Fig. 4.10a–d.** In this 23 year old patient with an electrophysiologically confirmed cone dystrophy one can see a central zone of atrophy (appearing in the FAF image as dark) surrounded by a ring of elevated FAF called a »rod ring«. This phenomenon, whose pathophysiological basis is not well understood, can also appear in patients with other hereditary retinal disorders, including retinitis pigmentosa and Leber's congenital amaurosis.

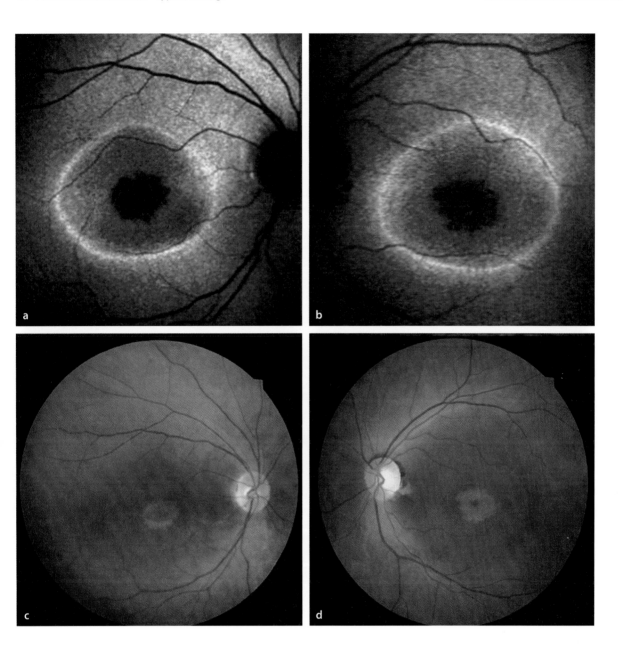

Macular Disorders

5.1   Age-Related Macular Degeneration (AMD)

Early and late stages of age related macular degeneration (AMD) can be identified. The early stages are characterized by retinal drusen and irregular pigmentation of the retinal pigment epithelium (RPE). The late stages have geographic atrophy of the RPE, RPE elevations, choroidal neovascularization and retinal angiomatous proliferation (RAP) as well as the formation of disciform scars.

5.1.1   Drusen

Drusen are deposits of protein and lipid containing material beneath the retinal pigment epithelium, usually accompanied by circumscribed areas of depigmentation or atrophy of the overlying RPE cells. Drusen are present in up to 80% of patients older than 60 years and are not specific for AMD. They are located in the posterior pole and are usually symmetrically distributed in both eyes. Drusen are differentiated as hard, soft and diffuse types. Retinal drusen, associated with the complex and multifactorial genesis of AMD, should be distinguished from so-called »juvenile« drusen, such as those found in cases of monogenic macular dystrophies.

Symptoms

Depending on the level of severity, isolated expression of drusen usually spares visual acuity for the most part, although difficulties with reading, color vision disturbances, mild metamorphopsia and delayed dark adaptation are usually present.

Fundus

Hard drusen appear as small, sharply defined and yellowish deposits beneath the RPE.

Soft drusen are larger sub-RPE deposits (soft drusen by definition have a diameter of more than 65 µm). These are less well defined and in later phases can merge with one another to produce circumscribed elevations of the RPE.

Diffuse drusen (also described as laminar drusen or cuticular drusen) are diffuse deposits beneath the RPE. Their appearance in electron microscopic images is used to further subdivide them into »basal laminar deposits« (deposits between the RPE-cell membrane and the RPE basal membrane) and »basal linear deposits« (deposits between the RPE-basal membrane and the remaining layers of Bruch's membrane). Diffuse drusen cannot be fully appreciated by their funduscopic appearance, although they can be accompanied by visible, yellowish, subretinal deposits.

Autofluorescence

In regions of drusen one can find unaltered, strongly elevated, or markedly diminished levels of autofluorescence. Large, soft drusen in particular are associated with areas of abnormal autofluorescence

Fluorescein angiography

Angiographic phenomena in the presence of drusen are affected by the status of the overlying RPE and the chemical composition of the drusen themselves. RPE atrophy over the drusen makes the choroidal background fluorescence more easily visible (so-called window defects). Drusen light up early in the angiogram, as the choroidal vessels fill. They are more easily recognizable during the angiogram than they are funduscopically. Large, soft drusen can mask the background fluorescence, meaning that the drusen material can be so extensive and dense that despite the presence of RPE defects, the background fluorescence can't be seen. In the late phase the angiographic appearance of drusen depends on their chemical composition and their corresponding affinity for hydrophilic dyes. A higher proportion of phospholipid favors binding of the fluorescein to the drusen, which are then hyperfluorescent (»staining«). Consequently, soft drusen are initially hypo- and then later hyper-fluorescent.

Diffuse drusen have a fluorescein angiographic appearance described as »stars in the sky«: countless numbers of uniform, round hyperfluorescent spots (window defects).

To the extent that vitelliform material is present, the background fluorescence will be blocked in the early phase, followed by a late staining effect.

ICG-Angiography

Analogous to fluorescein angiography and depending on their chemical composition,, drusen can bind to ICG, causing hyperfluorescence in the late phase (the »staining phenomenon«). The chemical composition of drusen may depend on their etiology and the age of the patient. ICG-staining is particularly common in younger patients.

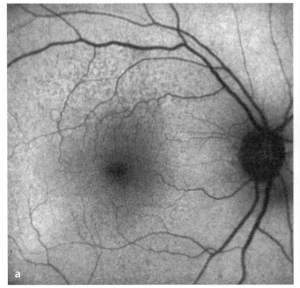
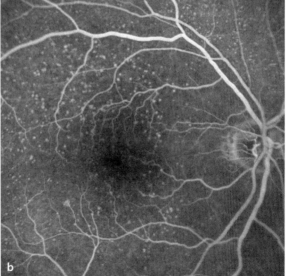

◘ **Fig. 5.1a,b.** A 74 year old patient with hard drusen in the right eye, acuity 20/25. **a** Autofluorescence. A few drusen, particularly above the macula, are marked by a reduced autofluorescence signal, causing an irregular pattern of fluorescence in this area. Other types of drusen do not alter the autofluorescence signal. **b** During fluorescence angiography the drusen appear as hyperfluorescent without any indication of leakage in the late phase.

■ **Fig. 5.2a–d.** A 24 year old patient with juvenile drusen that were incidentally discovered at age 5. Acuity 20/20 in both eyes with no visual problems. **a** Fundus appearance of the right eye. **b,c** Fluorescein angiography of the right eye: the drusen appear hyperfluorescent with increasing intensity during the course of the study. **d** Fluorescein angiography of the left eye shows an identical appearance.

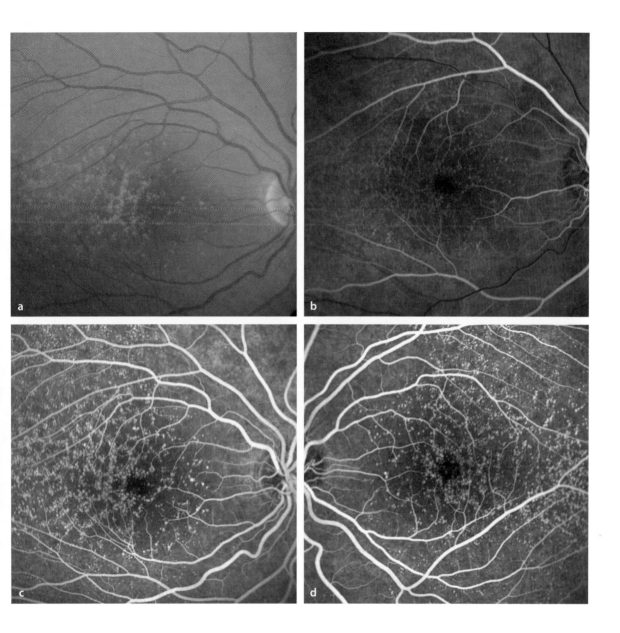

Fig. 5.3a–f. A 70 year old patient with confluent soft drusen. **a,b** Fundus and autofluorescence findings in the right eye. The drusen are hypofluorescent in the early phase and become progressively hyper-fluorescent from uptake of the fluorescein during the course of the study. **f** ICG-angiography: Since the drusen don't take up the ICG, they are not detectable during the study

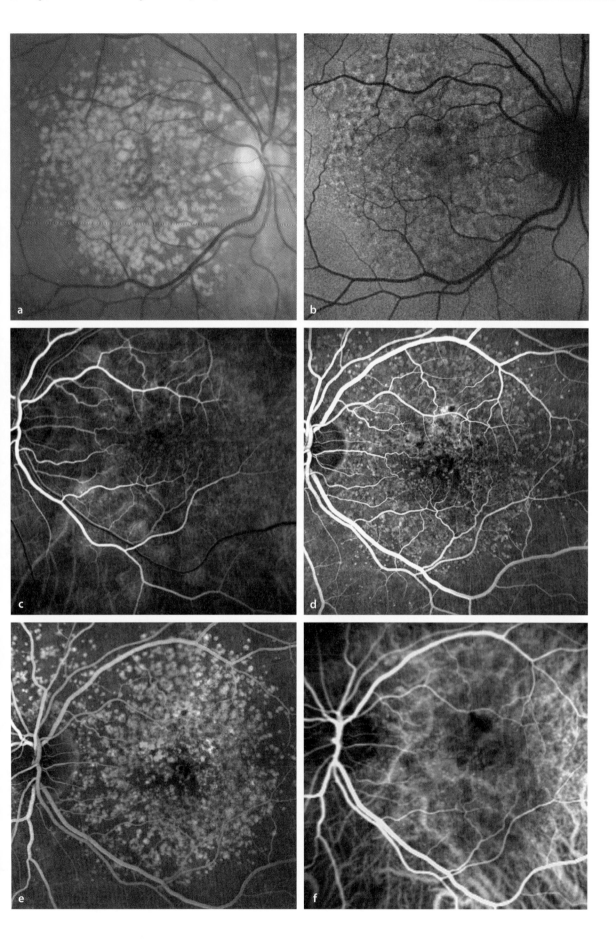

5.1.2 Irregular Pigmentation of the Retinal Pigment Epithelium (RPE)

Circumscribed hyper- or hypopigmentation of the RPE can be an early sign of age-dependent macular degeneration, but is not a specific finding. It can be found in association with many different disorders. Hyperpigmentation can arise by proliferation and clumping of RPE cells on top of one another or by increasing melanin content of individual cells. Also, hyperpigmentation can occur at the level of the neurosensory retina by in migration of RPE cells and/or macrophages containing melanin. RPE hypopigmentation can appear independently of drusen formation, either by reduced pigment content or by loss of RPE cells.

Symptoms

Symptoms depend on the location of the changes, the underlying disease process, and the sequence of alterations to the RPE. Most are of limited functional relevance.

Fundus

Irregular areas of hypo- and hyperpigmentation in the posterior pole.

Fluorescein Angiography

Areas of hypopigmentation appear hyperfluorescent, due to transmission of the background choroidal fluorescence (window defect). Areas of hyperpigmentation block the background fluorescence, and appear as hypofluorescent. An angiographic study is necessary only if the clinical evaluation suggests the possibility of choroidal neovascularization (see below).

5.1.3 Geographic atrophy of the RPE

RPE atrophy is seen as flat, atrophic areas of the RPE and the outer retinal layers, including the photoreceptor layer, and the choriocapillaris. It can appear as the primary manifestation of AMD or as a secondary sign of progression of other stages of AMD, including drusen, RPE detachment, or choroidal neovascularization.

Symptoms

Symptoms are those of scotomas corresponding to affected retinal areas.

Fundus

Flat areas of hypopigmentation with sharply defined margins. Due to atrophy of the choriocapillaris in these areas, the large choroidal vessels are visible.

Autofluorescence

Atrophy of the RPE extinguishes the autofluorescence phenomenon, and areas of geographic atrophy appear hypofluorescent. In the border zones of geographic atrophy the cells of the RPE have an elevated content of lipofuscin, which leads to a marked increase in autofluorescence at the margins of areas of geographic atrophy (▶ Chapter 4).

Fluorescein Angiography

One sees the hyperfluorescence of window defects. Depending on the extent of the accompanying atrophy of the choriocapillaris, the larger choroidal vessels will be visible.

◘ **Fig. 5.5a–d.** Geographic atrophy of the RPE, left eye. **a** Fundus appearance. **b** Extinction of autofluorescence in the atrophic area. Surrounding the atrophic zone is a band of increased hyperfluorescence, correlating to the accumulated lipofuscin content of the RPE cells. **c** The same patient one year later: In areas of elevated lipofuscin storage, one can see the formation of additional, smaller zones of atrophy. **d** The same patient another year later: increasing spread and coalescence of the zones of geographic atrophy.

Fig. 5.4. Geographic atrophy of the RPE. Fluorescein angiography shows a sharply margined central area of transmission of the choroidal vascular fluorescence. In the course of the angiogram there is no change in the size of the hyperfluorescent border zone and no leakage.

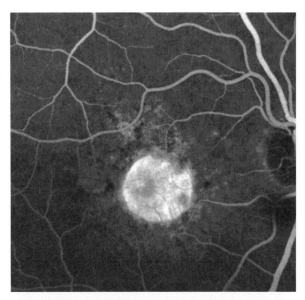

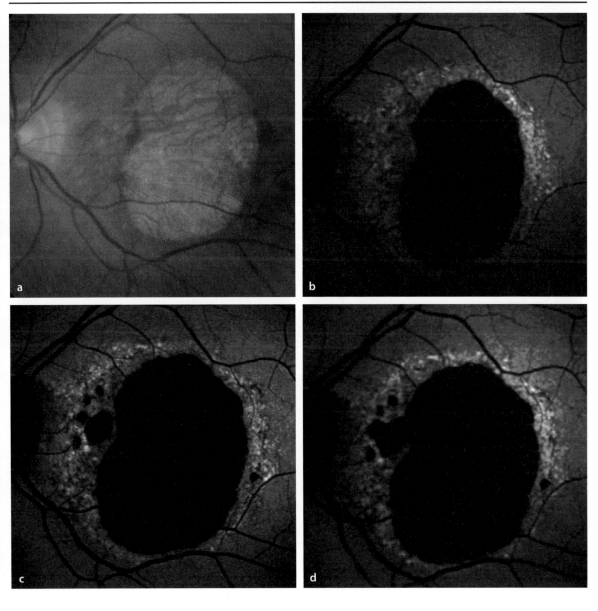

5.1.4 Choroidal Neovascularization (CNV)

Choroidal neovascularization (CNV) is the formation of vascular budding in the choriocapillaris. Neovascularization is classified as: Type 1, vessels spreading between the choriocapillaris and the RPE (◨ Fig. 5.6a), and Type 2, vessels that have grown through the RPE to lie between the RPE and the neurosensory retina (◨ Fig. 5.6b). During growth, the CNV vessels of Type 1 can cause formation of multiple wrinkles in the RPE, eventually surrounding the RPE on all sides. Neovascular membranes growing beneath the RPE can cause fibrovascular detachments. Mixed forms of types 1 and 2 are not uncommon.

Symptoms

Depending on the location of the choroidal neovascularization, there may be a marked reduction in visual acuity with metamorphopsia, a relative scotoma due to intraretinal, subretinal, and/or sub pigment epithelial exudation or bleeding

Fundus

Macular edema, exudates and hemorrhages. A classical CNV can appear as a circumscribed, reddish-gray subretinal area of altered funduscopic appearance.

Fluorescein Angiography

Based on the fluorescein angiographic appearance, choroidal neovascularization is classified as either the classic or the occult form. Not uncommonly, though, one can find both types (see below). In addition to the CNV itself, the AMD lesion can also have hemorrhages, exudates, pigmentation changes, or RPE detachments. Hence, the fluorescein angiographic appearance of neovascular AMD can be highly variable, and the individual components of the collective lesion are difficult to classify.

5.1.4.1 Classic Choroidal Neovascularization

So-called »classic« choroidal neovascularization is mostly located between the RPE and the neurosensory retina (Type 2, see above), and is more easily defined by angiography than is occult CNV.

Fluorescein Angiography

Classic choroidal neovascular membranes are visible already at the onset of the early angiographic phase. CNV lesions have hyperfluorescent borders, due to a higher density of vessels in these regions, and can also be surrounded by outer zones of hypofluorescence, making them easily seen. Frequently, individual vessels within the membrane are identifiable, usually by virtue of the »wagon wheel« pattern they form. This pattern is made up of central vessels that supply the blood, and the centripetally oriented vessels that radiate from the center. During the course of the angiographic study, a marked leakage from the vascular membrane becomes evident, which causes the margins of the membrane to become increasingly indistinct. In the late phase one finds diffuse leakage spread over a broad area.

ICG Angiography

ICG angiography reveals the vascular networks of classic CNV lesions. A hypofluorescent outer border can surround the CNV. Since 98% of ICG is bound to albumin, there has to be a markedly reduced vascular barrier function, before ICG can leak from a CNV membrane. With the assistance of ICG angiography, one can frequently identify the »feeder vessel« that supplies blood to the CNV membrane. This is clinically important, since a targeted photocoagulation of the feeder vessel can lead to an involution of the entire membrane.

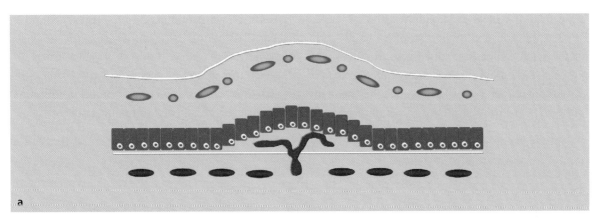

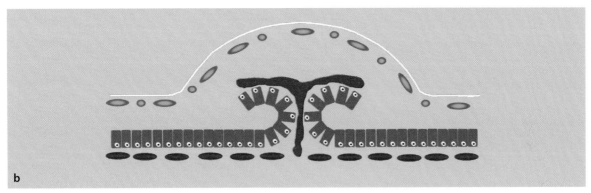

Fig. 5.6a,b

▣ **Fig. 5.7a–f.** A 74 year old patient with classic CNV. Funduscopic **a** and autofluorescent **b** images show relatively subtle changes superior to the fovea. Fluorescein angiography **c–e** demonstrates a sharply bordered area of hyperfluorescence in the early phase with a surrounding zone of hypofluorescence. Hyperfluorescent borders are not usually found in classic CNV lesions. In the late phase of the study **e** is typical leakage of dye. The vertical OCT (Optical Coherence Tomography) section shows the small subretinal CNV (*arrow*), as well as a bordering subretinal accumulation of fluid and intraretinal edema.

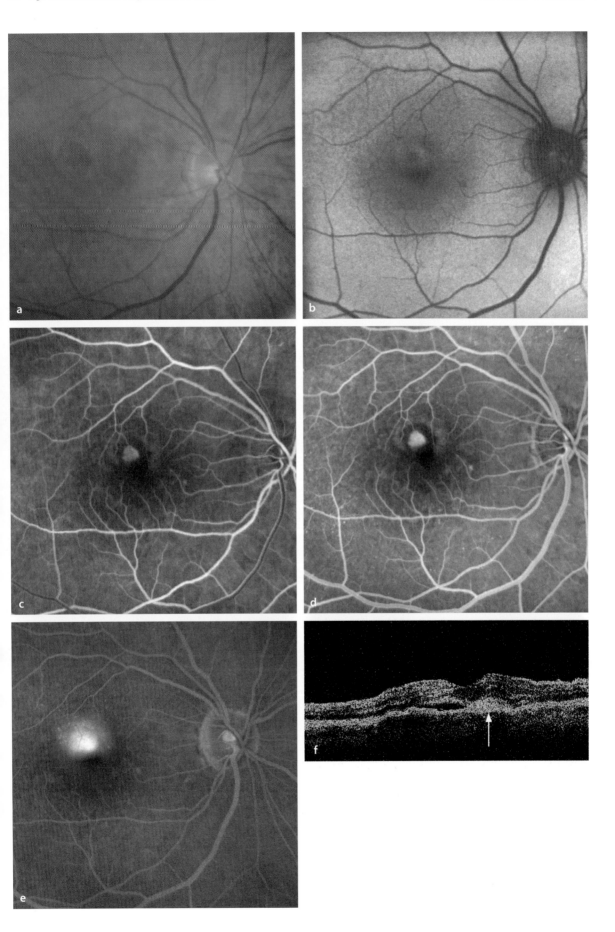

5

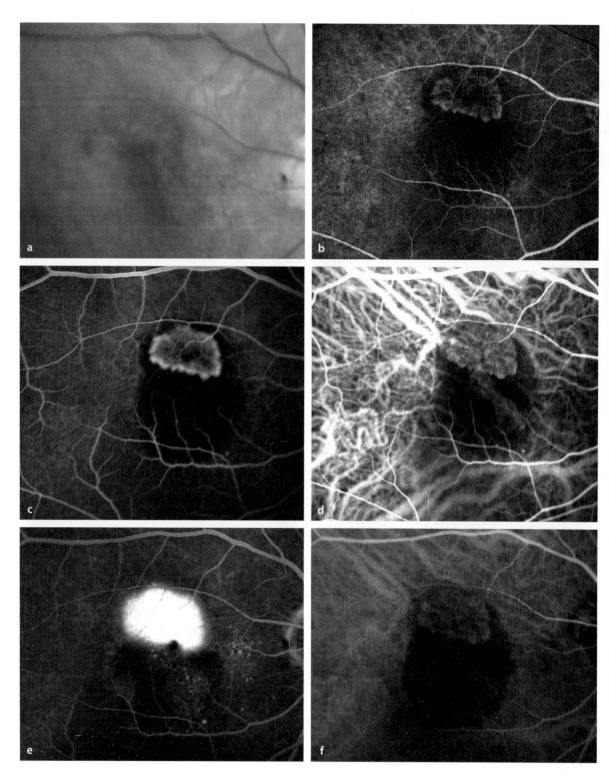

■ **Fig. 5.8a–f.** A 70 year old patient with AMD. **a** Fundus appearance. **b,c** Fluorescein angiography demonstrates a classic CNV in the early phase with a well demarcated area of hyperfluorescence and a hypofluorescent surrounding zone. Inferior to the CNV is a circumscribed blockage of the background fluorescence, caused by a hemorrhage, making the CNV stand out in high contrast. In the simultaneous ICG angiogram **d** the spoked wheel pattern of the CNV vascular network is easily recognizable. In the late phase **e** there is a heavy leakage of fluorescein, which reaches beyond the border of the CNV, but no leakage of ICG **f**.

5.1.4.2 Occult Choroidal Neovascularization

Occult choroidal vascular membranes lie beneath the RPE (between the choriocapillaris and the RPE, Type 1, see above). They are surrounded by RPE, making them difficult to distinguish from unaffected regions, hence the term »occult«. Occult forms make up about 80% of all newly diagnosed CNV, making them far more common than the classic form. Occult choroidal neovascular lesions can grow through the RPE, transforming them from Type 1 to Type 2 lesions.

Fluorescein Angiography

Traditionally, two different forms of occult CNV have been differentiated based on their angiographic appearance: fibrovascular RPE detachment, and late stage leakage of indeterminate origin. This differentiation goes back to the original Macular Photocoagulation Study (MPS), conducted in the late 1980's and early 1990's, when these terms were introduced as definitions in the study's design. Generally, it can be said that occult CNV lesions have no directly identifiable vessels, giving only indirect clues to their presence. Thus in the early phase of the angiogram there are either no or only limited indications of hyperfluorescence. In the course of the angiogram. there is a slowly increasing, irregular hyperfluorescence with leakage of dye in the late phase. These regions of hyperfluorescence do not correlate with drusen or zones of RPE atrophy. Usually, the source of the leakage cannot be identified in the early phase of the study.

Fibrovascular RPE Detachment

RPE detachments are produced when an occult CNV causes irregular elevation of the RPE, which can be particularly well seen when examining stereoscopic image pairs. This elevation becomes apparent about 1-2 minutes into the angiogram as an area of irregularly stippled hyperfluorescence that is much weaker than the hyperfluorescence of a classic CNV. The hyperfluorescence increases steadily into the late phase of the study, producing a flat area of hyperfluorescence that marks the region of the fibrovascular RPE detachment. The borders of the detachment are often indistinct, since the fluorescence intensity at the edge of the elevated RPE can be irregular, fading at varying rates. Also, the smooth transition from the attached to the detached area of RPE contributes to the poor definition of its edges. Fibrovascular RPE detachments must be distinguished from purely serous RPE detachments (see below).

Late Leakage of Undetermined Origin

This type of occult CNV is less commonly diagnosed than is the fibrovascular RPE detachment. In this form there is no clinically identifiable RPE detachment and the functional impairment of vision is usually less, since it produces a more limited degree of exudation. A few minutes after the fluorescein injection, an inhomogeneous, irregular area of hyperfluorescence appears and gradually increases in intensity into the late phase of the study. At the corresponding location during the early phase there is no specific location of hyperfluorescence that can be identified as the source.

ICG Angiography

Occult CNV lesions show a variable pattern during ICG angiography. »Hot spots« are well defined foci of ICG hyperfluorescence located within the same area as the occult CNV, as defined by the fluorescein angiogram. They become increasingly recognizable during the mid to late phases of the ICG angiogram. These hot spots can represent active CNV lesions, they can arise from idiopathic polypoid choroidal vasculopathy, or they can mark the presence of a retinal angiomatous proliferation (see below). Hot spots are smaller than the area of the optic disc. ICG plaques of hyperfluorescence on the other hand are by definition areas of hyperfluorescence that are larger than the optic disc. Such plaques are evident in the late phase of the study. In occult CNV lesions they can also reveal the feeder vessels during the ICG angiographic study (see above).

■ **Fig. 5.9a–f.** A 72 year old patient with occult choroidal neovascularization and detachment of the retinal pigment epithelium in the left eye. With stereoscopic fundus imaging one sees irregular elevation of the retinal pigment epithelium, which is not visibly identifiable by conventional fundus photography **a**. During fluorescein angiography in the early phase **b** there is at first a loss of background fluorescence. Not until a few minutes later is an irregular area of hyperfluorescence apparent, with no indication of its point of origin. In the late phase **e** there is a distinct area of leakage with pooling of the fluorescent dye beneath the RPE detachment. An OCT section running from 7 to 1 o'clock (from lower nasal to upper temporal) shows several fibrovascular detachments of the RPE **f**.

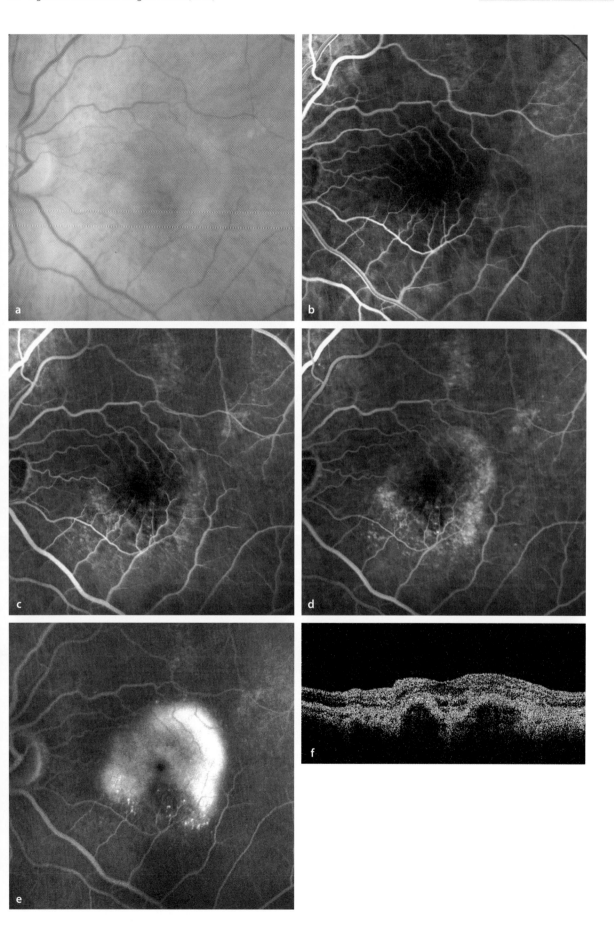

5

Fig. 5.10a–f. A 78 year old patient with progressive loss of acuity and metamorphopsia in the left eye. In the right eye an AMD lesion has already reached the cicatricial stage. **a** Fundoscopy finds central, irregularly pigmented lesions, elevations of the RPE and cystoid macular edema. **b** Autofluorescence shows the collective size of the pathological process, which by its irregular autofluorescence is clearly distinguishable from the physiological, homogeneous autofluorescence of the surrounding fundus. **c, d** Fluorescein angiography at first finds a reduction of background fluorescence, followed by an increasingly bright and diffuse area of hyperfluorescence. **e** In the late phase a very pronounced accumulation of cystoid macular edema is apparent. **f** An OCT section through the lesion shows an irregular course of the RPE and an area of advanced cystoid macular edema with an occult CNV.

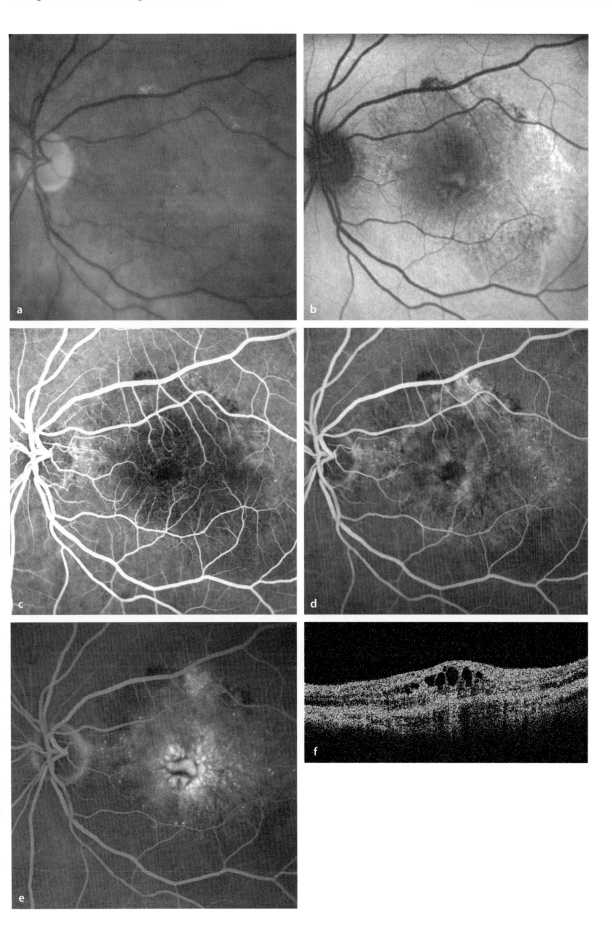

5.1.4.3 Mixed Forms

The terms »classic« and »occult« describe fluorescein angiographic patterns and are not absolutely associated with good or poor discrimination of a CNV membrane (an occult membrane in a few cases can also have well defined angiographic borders). Frequently, mixed forms of angiographic patterns are apparent. When a CNV membrane is called predominantly classic, it is meant that more than 50% of the CNV has a classic angiographic pattern. A CNV with »minimally classic choroidal neovascularization« describes a membrane with angiographic characteristics of the classic form in less than 50% of the entire CNV border.

5.1.4.4 Localization of Choroidal Neovascularization

Aside from typifying CNV as classic or occult, the precise location of the CNV membrane (par-ticularly for classic CNV) is clinically important. Location is also determined by fluorescein angiography. In addition to subfoveal lesions there are juxtafoveal CNV membranes (border of membrane within 1-199 μm of the center of the foveal avascular zone) and extrafoveal CNV membranes (margin at least 200 μm from the foveal center). During the Macular Photocoagulation Study (MPS), exact topographical localization was necessary for determining the need for intervention. With the advent of pharmacologic anti-VEGF therapies, however, this has become less relevant. The lesions of AMD may contain several of the various pathological components, such as CNVM (classic, occult or minimally classic), hemorrhages, subretinal fluid, and/or serous RPE detachment(s). For localization of a CNVM, however, the location of the lesion itself is decisive. An extrafoveal CNV can also be associated with an accumulation of subfoveal fluid (which becomes apparent in the late phase of a fluorescein angiogram).

Fig. 5.11a–c. a Extrafoveal CNV (in the papillomacular bundle). Fluorescein angiography (early phase, mid phase, late phase). **b** Juxtafoveal CNV. Fluorescein angiography (early phase, mid phase, late phase). **c** Subfoveal CNV. Fluorescein angiography (early phase, mid phase, late phase).

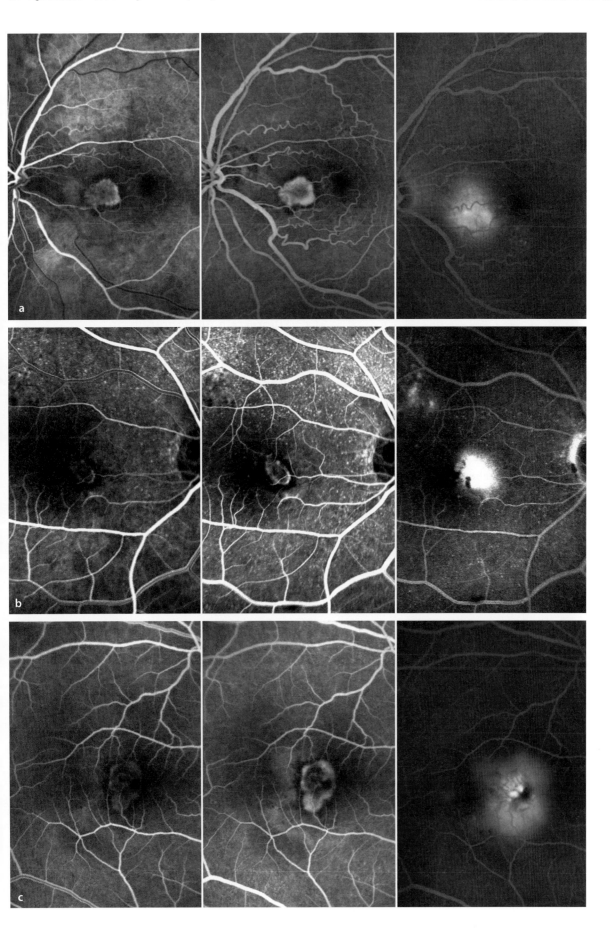

5.1.5 Serous Detachment of the Retinal Pigment Epithelium

Causes of an RPE detachment include: a fibrovascular membrane (fibrovascular RPE detachment, see occult CNV), a hemorrhage beneath the RPE, confluent large drusen (drusenoid RPE detachment), idiopathic polypoid choroidal vasculopathy (see below), retinal angiomatous proliferation (see below) or a purely exudative accumulation of fluid between Bruch's membrane and the RPE. The latter is called a serous RPE detachment. Serous detachments are thought to be formed when Bruch's membrane is altered by deposits that make it increasingly hydrophobic, which causes formation of a barrier to the normal flow of fluid from the retinal pigment epithelium cells into the choriocapillaris. Retinal pigment epithelium cells then pump fluid in the direction of the choriocapillaris, without it being able to flow sufficiently well through Bruch's membrane. The fluid collects under the RPE and with continued active pumping of fluid, the RPE is elevated above Bruch's membrane. RPE detachments can flatten out over time, or they can progress to formation of a break in the RPE. Another pathogenetic mechanism for a serous RPE detachment can be a small CNV membrane beneath the RPE that contributes to the RPE elevation. This can be very difficult to diagnose. Strictly speaking, this is a mixed form that includes both a serous RPE detachment and an additional fibrovascular RPE detachment. One speaks of a »vascular serous RPE detachment« (in contradistinction to an »avascular, serous RPE detachment«).

Fundus

A serous detachment appears as a roundish to oval, gray elevation. By fundoscopy it is usually not apparent whether one has a serous or a vascular detachment. The presence of blood within the detachment and/or an indented margin suggest a vascular form of detachment.

Autofluorescence

In the region of an RPE detachment the autofluorescence intensity can be unchanged, depressed or elevated, which is probably determined by the composition of the subepithelial fluid (the quantities and types of fluorophores).

Fluorescein Angiography

In the early phase there is blockage of the background fluorescence in the area of the RPE detachment. Then there is a gradual diffusion of fluorescein into the sub RPE space, staining the lesion. With fluorescein angiography the demarcation of choroidal vessels within the RPE detachment and the differentiation between avascular and vascular forms of RPE detachment is generally not possible. Indications of a CNV include hyperfluorescence at the margins of, or an uneven hyperfluorescence within the RPE detachment.

ICG Angiography

During ICG angiography, the RPE detachment in both the early and late phases appears hypofluorescent (dark disc). In some RPE detachments one can easily distinguish a vascular net or a circumscribed area of hyperfluorescence (hot spot) standing out against the surrounding hypofluorescence. With the help of ICG angiography a retinochoroidal anastomosis or a polypoidal choroidal vasculopathy can sometimes be identified (see below).

Fig. 5.12a–d. A 76 year old patient with an avascular serous RPE detachment (right eye). **a** Circular elevation of the RPE. **b** Autofluorescence imaging finds a corresponding, round area of reduced background autofluorescence. **c,d** Simultaneous fluorescein (left) and ICG (right) angiography shows a gradual, homogeneous filling of the RPE detachment with fluorescein, but not with ICG.

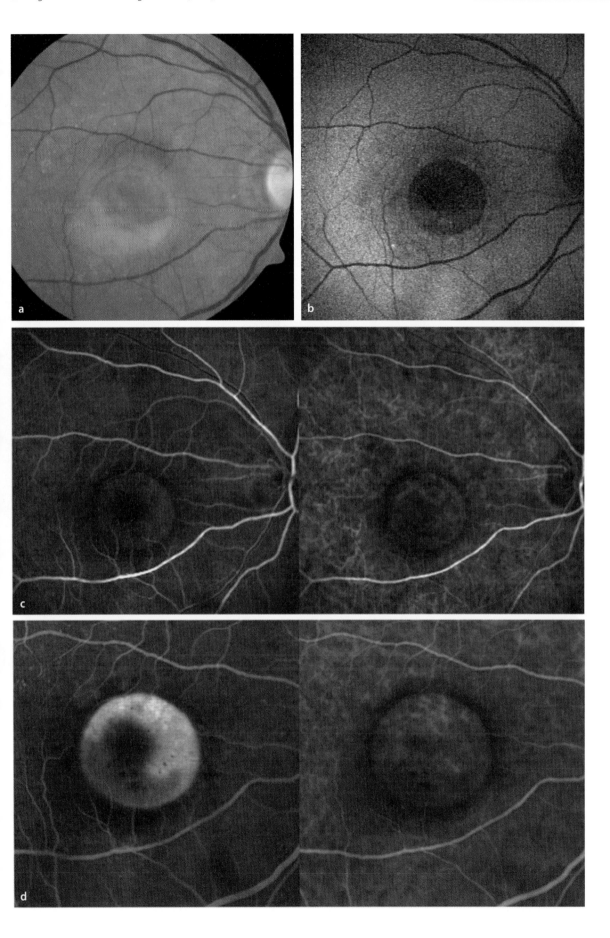

◨ **Fig. 5.13a–f.** A 78 year old patient with metamorphopsia in the right eye. **a** Fundus image shows a juxtafoveal, circumscribed area of increased pigmentation (RPE hypertrophy). Nasal to this area and extending into the infrafoveal macula, an RPE detachment extends to the fovea. **b** Autofluorescence shows an area of hyperfluorescence that correlates with the location of the RPE hypertrophy. The size of the lesion is made evident by the irregular zone of hyperfluorescence. The actual RPE detachment is marked by a subtle border of higher fluorescence, surrounded by a darker zone with subretinal fluid (*arrows* – compare to OCT image). **c,d** Fluorescein angiography shows an incomplete blockage of the background fluorescence at the locus of hyperpigmentation. **e** In the late phase one sees typical pooling of fluorescein beneath the RPE detachment, making its borders easily seen. **f** An OCT section through the detachment and extending from superotemporal to inferonasal shows its typical form. The detachment is surrounded by a slim border of subretinal fluid (*small star*).

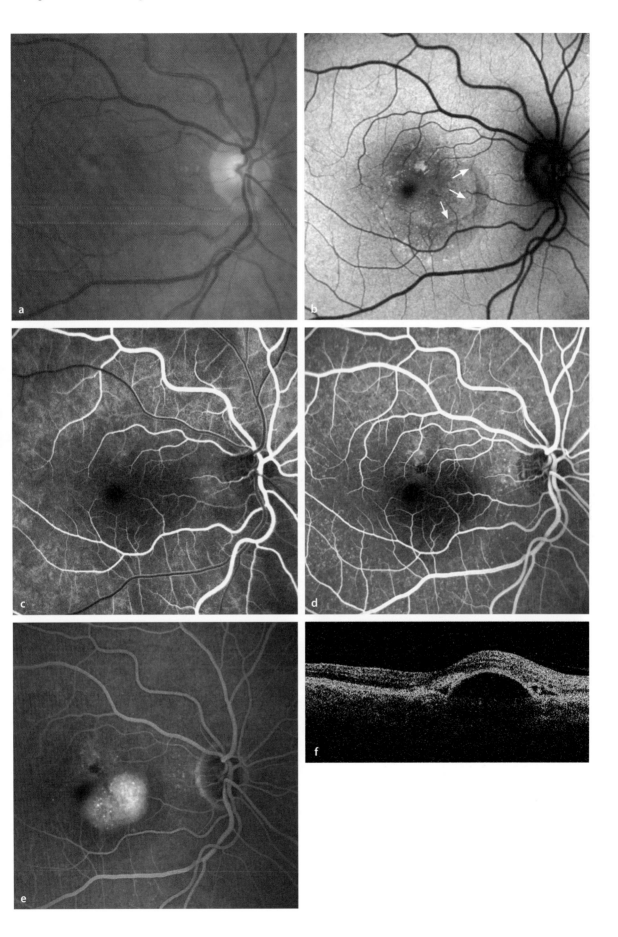

▣ Fig. 5.14a–d. Simultaneous fluorescein angiography (*left half images*) and ICG angiography (*right half images*) of a vascular serous RPE detachment (right eye). There is a central, circular RPE detachment marked by a round zone of hypofluorescence in both the fluorescein and ICG angiograms. Immediately in the early phase **a** near the border of the detachment, a zone of hyperfluorescence appears, indicating a focus of neovascularization. This is easily seen, is well demarcated, and is probably a patch of retinal angiomatous proliferation (RAP, ▶ Chapter 5.1.8). To what extent the neovascularization also lies within the choroid (CNV) cannot be determined with a certainty by angiography. During the course of the angiogram **b–d** there is increasing leakage from the neovascular tissue in the fluorescein angiogram, while in the ICG angiogram only the vascular net is seen. In the late phase **d** there is increasing pooling of fluorescein beneath the RPE detachment, while by contrast the RPE detachment in the ICG angiogram is only indirectly marked by persistent blockage of the background ICG fluorescence.

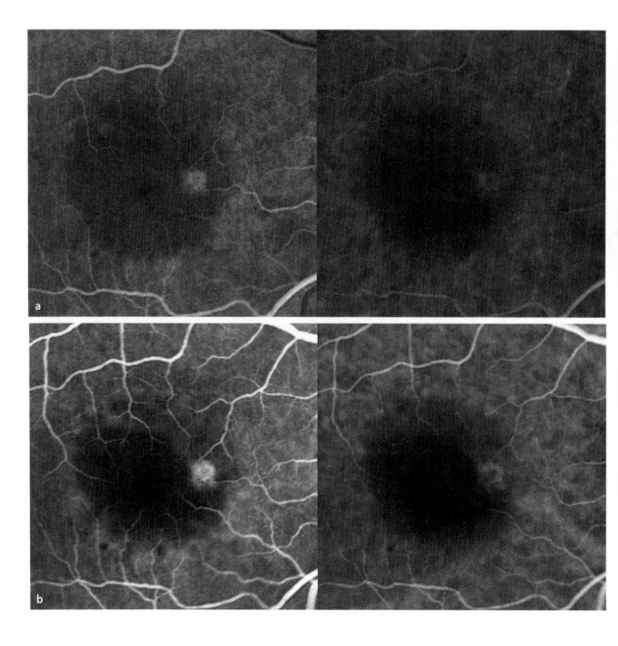

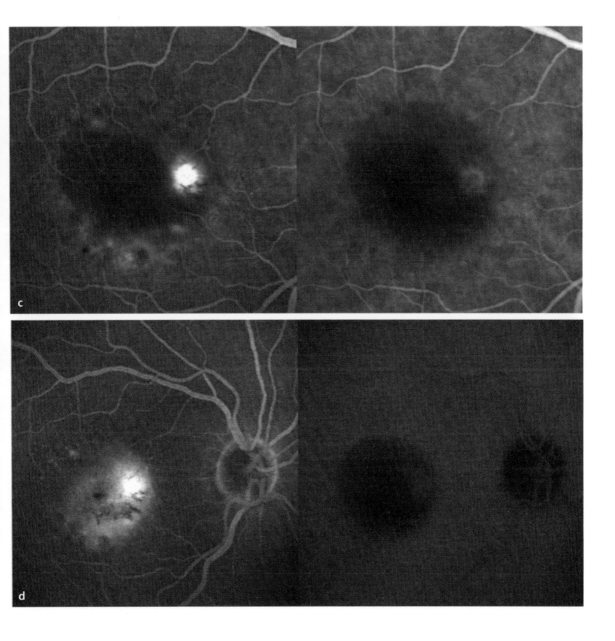

5.1.6 Breaks in the Retinal Pigment Epithelium (RPE)

As a rule, RPE breaks develop in the presence of an RPE detachment. RPE breaks are frequently accompanied by hemorrhages and abrupt losses of vision.

Fundus

RPE breaks can lead to subretinal hemorrhages, which makes assessment of the lesions more difficult. The lacerated RPE retracts, as a rule, so that there is often a sharply defined area in which the RPE is missing. Nearby, one frequently sees the torn, rolled up RPE as a brownish subretinal prominence.

Autofluorescence

In the areas where the RPE and its lipofuscin content are absent, there is no longer any retinal autofluorescence

Fluorescence Angiography

In areas where the RPE is missing the choroidal fluorescence shines through. If the RPE has retracted and curled, the thickened layer of RPE cells (having more than the normal unicellular thickness) blocks the background fluorescence. Subretinal hemorrhages likewise lead to areas of blocked fluorescence.

Fig. 5.15a–f. A 78 year old patient with sudden loss of vision in the left eye. **a** Fundoscopy shows a sharp margined, pale yellow area within the papillomacular bundle, within which the RPE has been torn away and is missing. In contradistinction to RPE defects of other origins (e.g. geographic RPE atrophy) the choroidal fluorescence is not visible. The pale yellow area suggests the presence of a fibrovascular membrane that initially caused an RPE detachment and then subsequently led to a break in the RPE. Beneath the break is a subretinal hemorrhage. The RPE in the papillomacular region is torn and has retracted and curled towards the fovea. This has produced an area near the fovea that has multiple layers of RPE, as indicated by the hyperpigmentation at its center. **b** In areas where the RPE is no longer present, the autofluorescence phenomenon is extinguished. **c–e** Angiographic fluorescence is visible in the area of the RPE break. The torn borders are sharply defined. The leakage in the late phase **e** suggests that a CNV membrane is present. **f** OCT imaging demonstrates an RPE detachment with an inwardly curled margin.

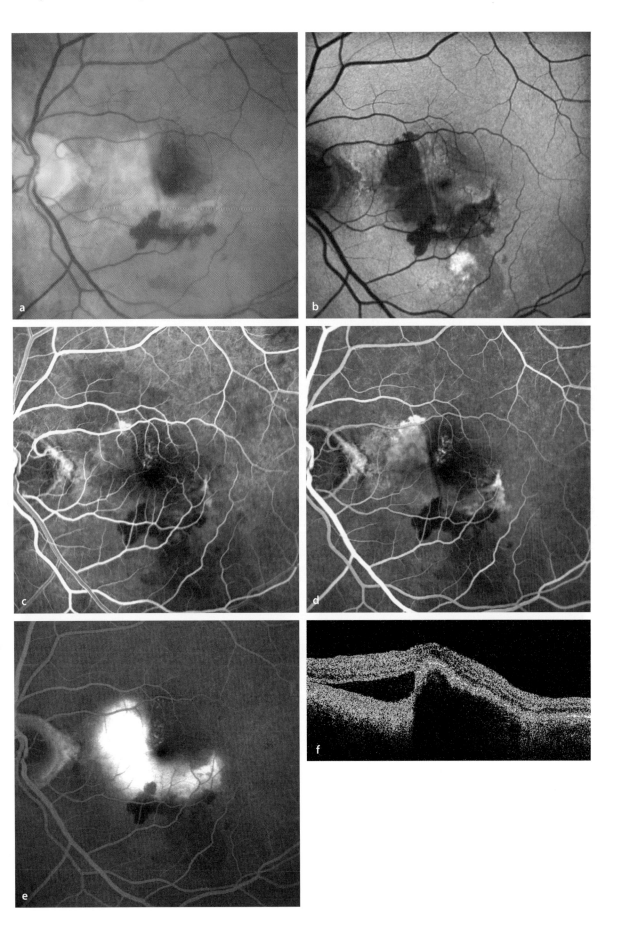

5.1.7 Idiopathic Polypoid Choroidal Vasculopathy

Idiopathic, polypoid, choroidal vasculopathy (IPCV) is a circumscribed lesion of the choroid, usually located at the temporal border of the optic disc or less frequently in the macula. It is an area of the choroid with a pathologically branched vascular net that has multiple (polyp shaped) areas of expansion. Hemorrhages and exudates are associated with these polypoidal vascular lesions. Consequently, RPE detachments often arise in the same locations. This disorder is regarded by some authors as a variant of AMD and is thought to have a higher frequency among patients of Asian and African origin than among those of European origin.

Fundus

Polypoid choroidal vascular ectasias are clinically recognizable as red-orange papules. There are also subretinal exudates, smaller RPE detachments and hemorrhages

Fluorescein Angiography

In the course of a fluorescein angiogram there is usually some leakage in the affected area.

ICG Angiography

ICG angiography is the optimal study for IPCV, since the vascular ectasias are well demonstrated without being masked by overlying exudation, as the case may be with fluorescein angiograms.

■ Fig. 5.16a–f. A 78 year old patient with gradual loss of visual acuity in the left eye to 20/50. a Fundoscopy shows an area of subretinal fluid bordering the temporal margin of the optic disc. Also, on the temporal margin of this area are hard exudates that reach all the way to the fovea. Stereoscopic examination of the area just temporal to the disc margin disclosed a deep, reddish papule (not visible in the fundus photo). b ICG angiography reveals circumscribed choroidal ectasias in the parapapillary zone that in the later course of the study d become more prominent. Fluorescein angiography of the parapapillary zone c,e demonstrates diffuse, progressive leakage of fluid. In the late phase of the ICG f a slow leakage of fluid is visible in the region of the vascular ectasias. The hard exudates block the ICG fluorescence, making them easily seen. The image pairs c and d as well as e and f are simultaneous image pairs taken from a combined fluorescein/ICG angiographic study.

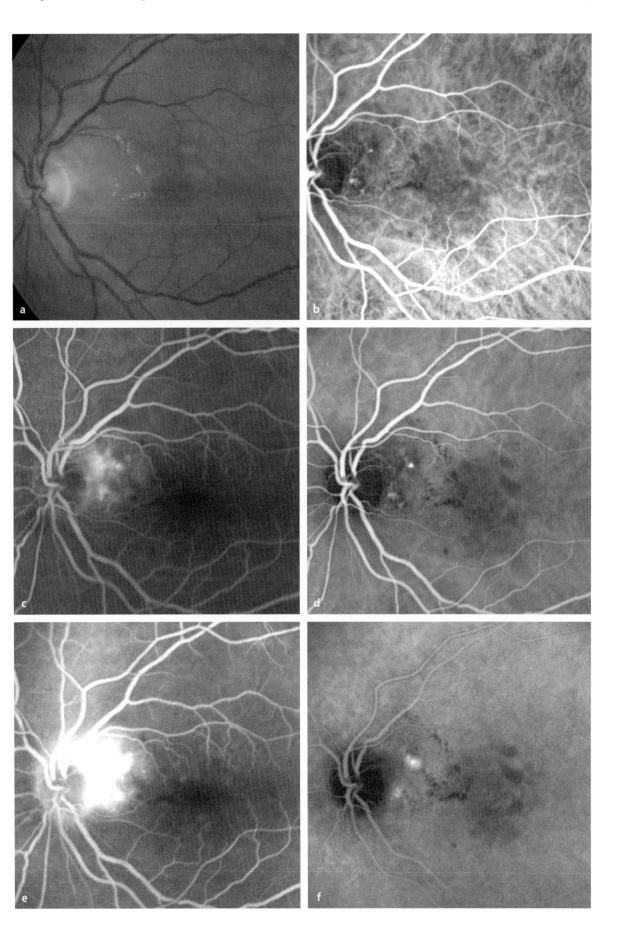

5.1.8 Retinal Angiomatous Proliferation (RAP)

Retinal angiomatous proliferation is a particular form of neovascular (exudative) AMD in which the neovascular process originates not in the choroid, but in the retina. There is a proliferation of retinal capillaries, formation of anastomoses between retinal arterioles and retinal venules, intraretinal neovascularization with development of angiomatous tissue components in the middle and deep layers of the retina, and finally formation of retinochoroidal anastomoses. In the late stage of development, neovascularization can also arise within the choroid (CNV). The retinochoroidal anastomoses of RAP should be distinguished from chorioretinal anastomoses, which develop secondarily in the late stages of primary choroidal neovascularization. RAP can lead to an associated serous RPE detachment, and in the presence of a CNV can also lead to a fibrovascular RPE detachment in the late stages.

Fundus

Fundoscopy reveals small retinal hemorrhages, retinal edema, occasionally hard exudates, intraretinal and in some cases subretinal neovascularization, and arteriovenous retinal anastomoses. Some RPE detachments can be identified by fundoscopy alone. Depending on the severity, one can also see varying degrees of subretinal exudation and bleeding. Retinochoroidal anastomoses are very difficult to recognize by fundoscopy alone.

Fluorescein Angiography

During the course of a fluorescein angiogram areas with retinal angiomatous proliferation will have progressively rising levels of leaked dye. Whether the neovascularization lies completely within the retina and has no subretinal components cannot be reliably determined by fluorescein angiography. Observation of other criteria like anastomosis formation or retinal vessels that extend into deeper layers are therefore very important.

ICG Angiography

With the help of ICG angiography the intraretinal vascular complexes and their identities as components of the retinal vasculature can be confirmed. ICG angiography can therefore contribute significantly to the study of RAP lesions.

Fig. 5.17a–h. A 58 year old patient with reduced acuity in the right eye and retinal angiomatous proliferation (RAP). **a** Fundoscopy. Small central retinal hemorrhages, surrounded by a zone of retinal edema (brighter round area). A retinal arteriole enters this area at 6 o'clock and then dives downward. A retinal venule arises at 12 o'clock and likewise turns towards deeper levels. **b** Fundus autofluorescence shows areas of masking that correlate with the locations of retinal hemorrhages. **c–h** Fluorescein angiography: initially, filling of the retinal arterial circulation. Then, appearance of a central, circumscribed intraretinal, nearly round lesion, which is probably fed by the retinal arteriolar vessel at 6 o'clock. Progressive filling of the venous circulation. **f** The central, intraretinal vascular complex is clearly recognizable. **g** Due to masking by a central hemorrhage, the vascular complex appears as a ring. **h** Finally, in the late phase there is clearly leakage of dye from the vascular complex.

5.1 · Age-Related Macular Degeneration (AMD)

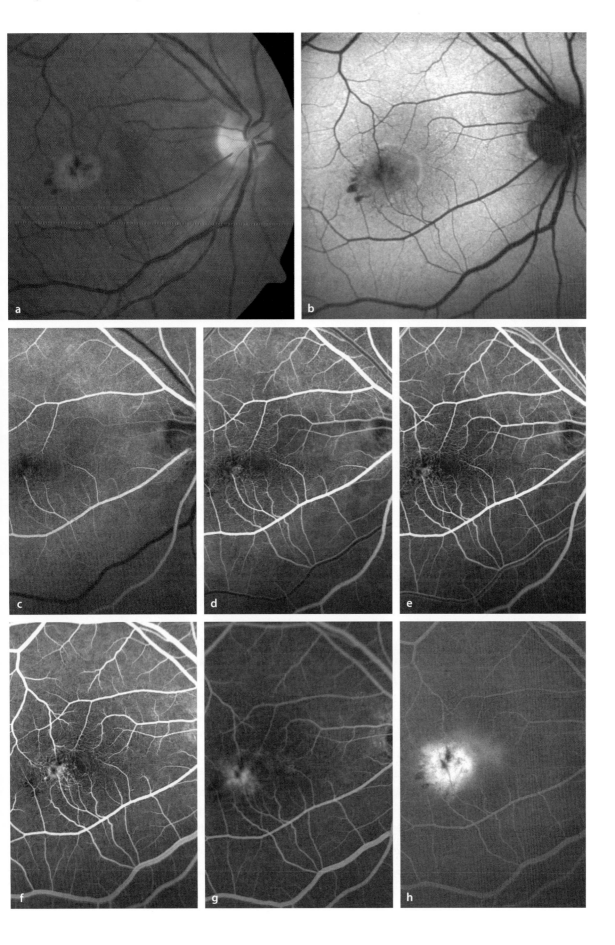

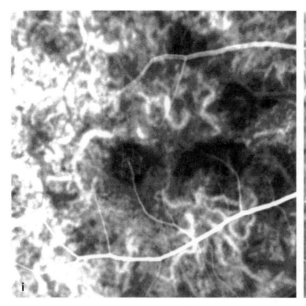
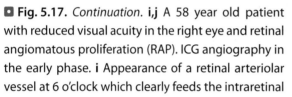
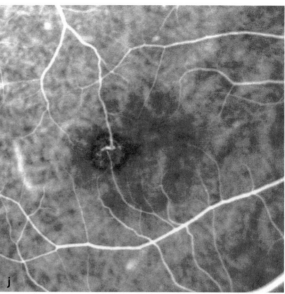

■ **Fig. 5.17.** *Continuation.* **i,j** A 58 year old patient with reduced visual acuity in the right eye and retinal angiomatous proliferation (RAP). ICG angiography in the early phase. **i** Appearance of a retinal arteriolar vessel at 6 o'clock which clearly feeds the intraretinal vascular complex. During the further course of the study, the retinal venular circulation is also clearly defined. **j** An anastomosis has formed between a retinal arteriole and a venule.

5.1.9 Disciform Scarring

The usual evolution of choroidal neovascularization concludes with the gradual formation of a fibrotic scar.

Fundus

A disciform scar appears - a fibrotic scarring of the choroidal vascular tissues. The photoreceptors in this area are destroyed. The clinical aspects of AMD in the cicatricial stage can be very different and depend on the size of the fibrotic zone, the original location of the choroidal neovascularization, the presence of atrophic areas of RPE and/or RPE clumping, and in some cases a persistent subretinal fluid and/or lipid exudation.

Autofluorescence

Within the area of scarring the autofluorescence phenomenon is extinguished.

Fluorescein Angiography

In the region of the fibrotic neovascular tissue a faint hyperfluorescence appears during fluorescein angiography that increases during the first minutes after the injection only to subsequently fade sway. If the hyperfluorescent areas of the early phase do not fade, there is likely to be some residual leakage of fluid.

ICG Angiography

Within the area of scarring one can often find anastomoses between the retinal and the choroidal vascular beds.

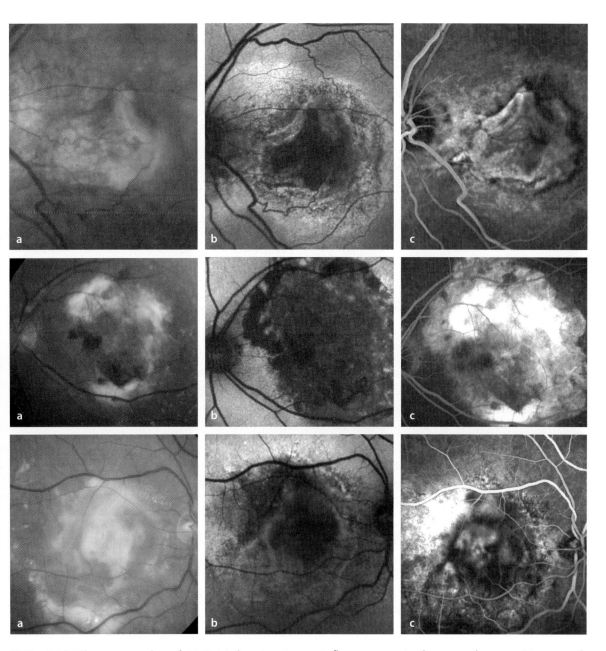

Fig. 5.18. Three examples of AMD in the cicatricial stage. **a** Fundoscopic findings. **b** Corresponding autofluorescence images with extinguishment of autofluorescence in the scarred area. **c** Corresponding fluorescein angiographic findings with staining of the cicatricial tissue.

5.1.10 Fluorescein Angiographic Phenomena Following Therapy

Neovascular AMD is managed with a number of therapeutic modalities, all of which rely on angiographic findings to judge the effects of therapy and the clinical course of disease.

5.1.10.1 Laser Coagulation

For classic extrafoveal CNV, conventional laser coagulation is usually successful (■ Fig. 5.19). The goal of therapy is to destroy the neovascular membrane, which must be monitored by means of fluorescein angiography. Any surviving portions of the membrane must be retreated by laser photocoagulation. This method has a high rate of relapse (up to 60%), during the first post-treatment year. As a rule the recurrence appears at the edge of the treated area closest to the fovea. Hot spots detected by ICG angiography and located in extrafoveal areas can also be managed by laser photocoagulation (■ Fig. 5.20). Extrafoveal feeder vessels detected by ICG angiography can also be treated by laser photocoagulation (■ Fig. 5.21). Since reappearance of the coagulated vessels is common, monitoring by ICG angiography is necessary.

5.1.10.2 Photodynamic Therapy (PDT)

The basic principle of PDT is the injection of a photosensitive substance, which is taken up by neovascular tissues in a relatively selective process, and subsequently activated by a non-thermal diode laser. This serves to set off a cascade of biological reactions, the consequence of which is to produce an intravascular thrombosis. This effect is frequently temporary only, so that a series of procedures is necessary, before a final closure of the CNV can be achieved.

Fundus

Following successful, usually multiple, sessions of PDT, the area of the CNV acquires a brownish pigmentation caused by the reactions of RPE cells. The neovascular process is then effectively stopped.

Fluorescein Angiography

PDT frequently results in decreased perfusion of the choriocapillaris in the treated area. This is a reversible which can be confirmed within a few weeks post treatment. Immediately following PDT of an area of CNV, there is often an increase in fluid leakage, but with successful destruction of the neovascular tissue, the leakage stops. A successfully treated focus of CNV can, much like the cicatricial stage of CNV, demonstrate staining (► Chapter 5.1.9). The inactivated neovascular membrane can acquire an uneven, drawn out border, and be larger than it was prior to treatment, but without resulting in a significant loss of vision (■ Fig. 5.22).

5.1.10.3 Anti VEGF Therapy

Intravitreal anti VEGF therapy with Ranibizumab, Bevacizumab or Pegaptanib can block the effects of the vascular growth factor VEGF, resulting in a decrease in vascular permeability and a reduction in fluid leakage from the newly formed vessels. With inhibition of the stimulus for neovascularization, the neovascular membrane is placed in a long-term state of inactivity. Similar to the events following PDT, the inactive CNV may become larger than it was prior to treatment, but without necessarily being accompanied by any deterioration in visual function (■ Fig. 5.24).

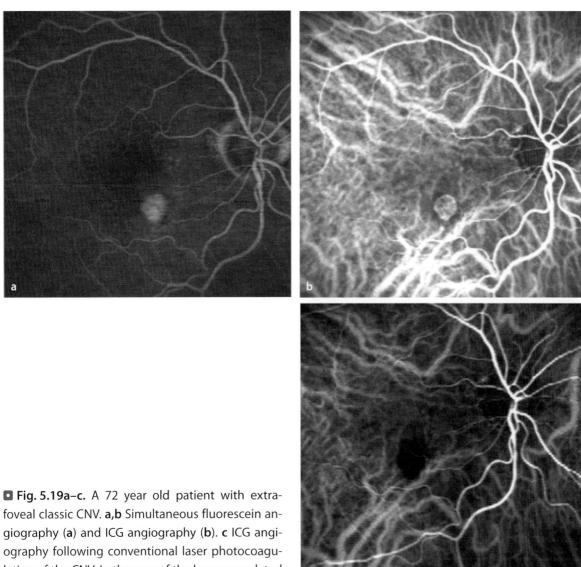

◘ **Fig. 5.19a–c.** A 72 year old patient with extra-foveal classic CNV. **a,b** Simultaneous fluorescein angiography (**a**) and ICG angiography (**b**). **c** ICG angiography following conventional laser photocoagulation of the CNV. In the area of the laser coagulated tissue no persistent vessels are demonstrable.

⬛ **Fig. 5.20a–i.** A 68 year old patient with abrupt loss of vision in the left eye, caused by a subretinal hemorrhage. **a** Simultaneous fluorescein and ICG angiography **b,c** shows blocking of fluorescence corresponding to the hemorrhage. Since the hemorrhage lies beneath the retina, the retinal vessels are clearly visible. **d–f** One week after treatment with rt-PA (recombinant tissue plasminogen activator) and gas injection the hemorrhage has been shifted. While fluorescein angiography **c** gives no indication of the source, ICG angiography **e** demonstrates an extrafoveal »hot spot«, which was treated with conventional laser photocoagulation. **g–h** Following complete resorption of the blood, the acuity is 20/20. Angiographically the site of coagulation treatment is hypofluorescent, due to destruction of the choriocapillaris. **i** The »hot spot« is no longer visible during ICG angiography.

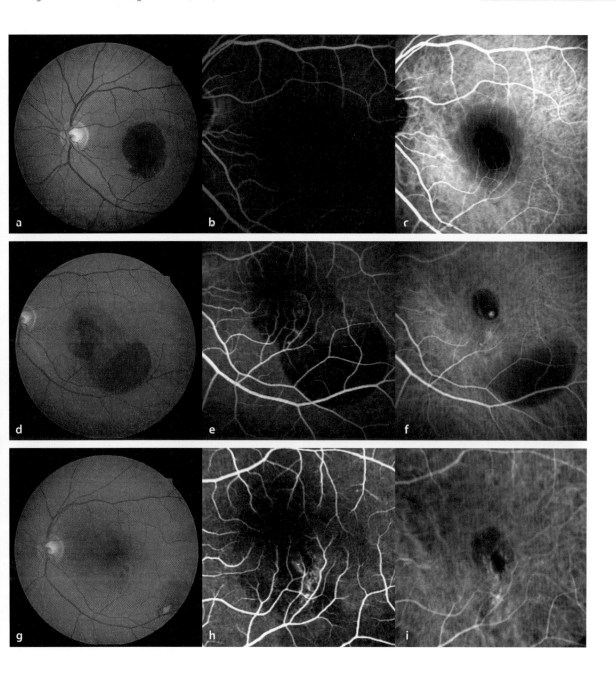

Fig. 5.21a–d. A 63 year old patient with peripapillary chorioretinal atrophic foci and acute metamorphopsia in the left eye. **a** Fundoscopy shows a central zone of subretinal fluid. **b** Fluorescein angiography reveals a classic subfoveal CNV lesion. **c** ICG angiography demonstrates a fan-shaped vascular pattern of CNV (*short arrows*) and a large choroidal vessel providing the blood supply (feeder vessel, *long arrows*). **d** Following laser coagulation of the feeder vessel, there has been a regression of the CNV. ICG angiography shows that both the feeder vessel and the neovascular membrane are no longer visible.

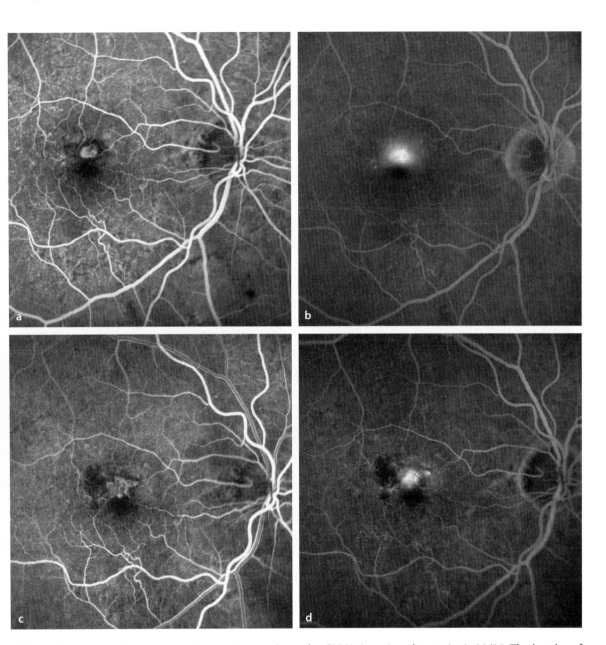

■ **Fig. 5.22a–d.** An 85 year old patient with juxtafo-veal classic CNV and an acuity of 20/50. a Fluorescein angiography shows the CNV to be well defined, and to have a narrow, surrounding border of hypofluo-rescence. **b** The late phase shows definite leakage of dye. **c** After four treatments with PDT one year later the CNV is inactive, the acuity is 20/25. The border of the CNV can be seen in the early phase of the fluo-rescein angiogram to be well defined and with an uneven margin. No leakage is seen during the study. In the late phase a small area of hyperfluorescence in the sense of »staining«.

Fig. 5.23a–f. A 72 year old patient, left eye. **a,b** Fluorescein angiography during a routine evaluation, acuity 20/20 in each eye. Below the fovea is an area of irregular pigmentation in the RPE with no leakage of dye. **c,d** Fluorescein angiography 1.5 years later. A juxtafoveal classic CNV has formed. The acuity has fallen to 20/30. **d** Leakage from the CNV in the late phase. **e,f** 3 months following PDT combined with an intravitreal injection of triamcinolone the CNV is no longer demonstrable by fluorescein angiography.

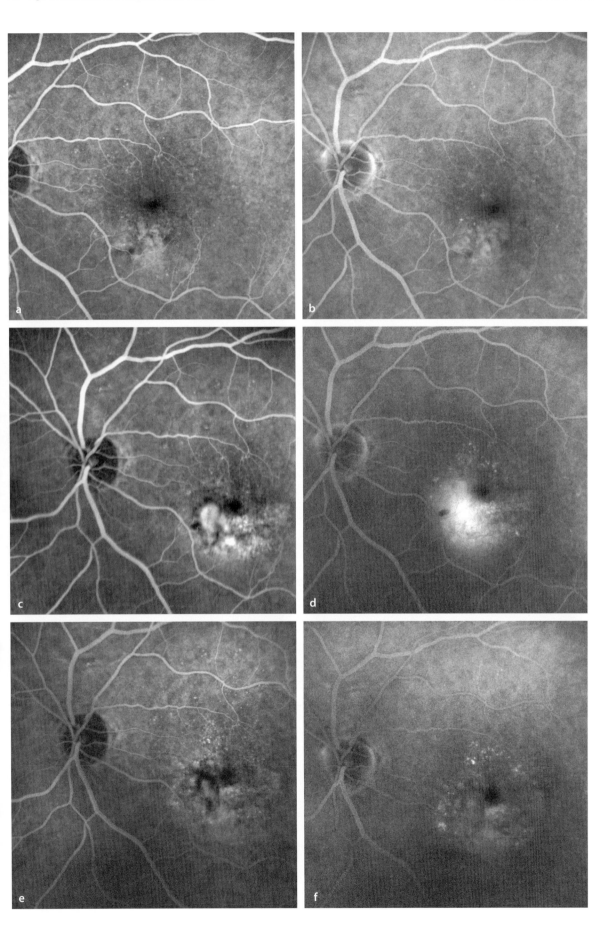

◨ **Fig. 5.24a–d.** A 77 year old patient with metamorphopsia and loss of acuity to 20/100 in the right eye. The fluorescein angiogram shows a classic subfoveal CNV with clearly defined leakage of dye in the late phase. **b** The patient received anti VEGF treatments (altogether 7 injections of intravitreal Pegaptanib in the course of one year). **c,d** One year later the CNV is inactive. Fluorescein angiography shows the CNV with irregular, drawn out, sharply defined margins without leakage in the late phase, acuity of 20/80

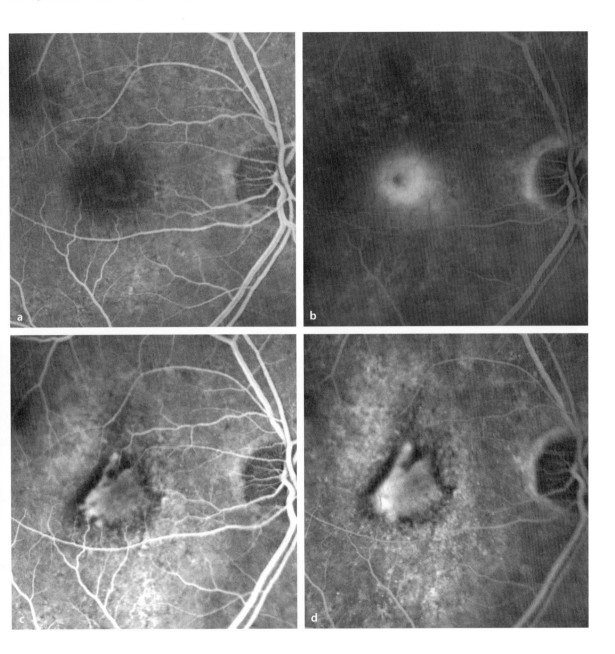

Fig. 5.25a–f. A 79 year old patient with reduced acuity and metamorphopsia in the right eye. **a** Fundoscopy reveals a subfoveal area of edema. Incidentaly noted are myelinated nerve fibers on the superior margin of the optic disc. **c,e** Fluorescein angiography shows a classic subfoveal CNV membrane with clear leakage of dye in the latephase **e**. The patient was treated with intravitreal injection of an anti-VEGF antibody and PDT. **b** Six weeks after treatment fundoscopy demonstrates no subretinal fluid. **d,f** The CNV membrane is no longer detectable by fluorescein angiography. In the late phase **f** there is no leakage.

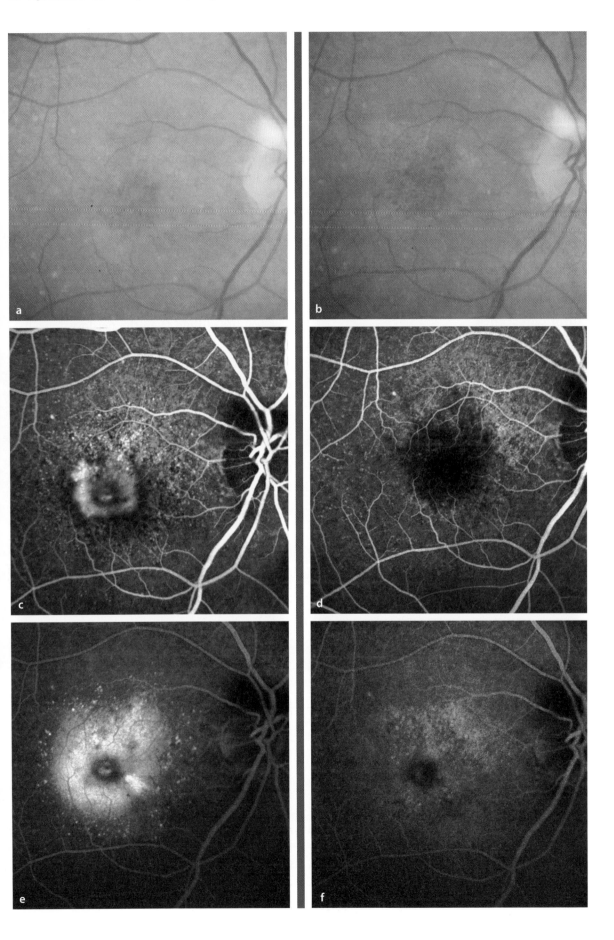

5.2   Cystoid Macular Edema

Cystoid macular edema (CME) originates in a disturbance of vascular permeability in the perifoveal capillaries and/or in the retinal pigment epithelium. CME appears as an accumulation of fluid in the outer plexiform layer of the retina (Henle's fiber layer), in which characteristic cyst-like fluid filled spaces form. It is a non-specific reaction of the macular tissues that can arise in association with many different disorders, including diabetic retinopathy, tributary retinal vein occlusions, uveitis, epiretinal membranes, and postoperatively following ophthalmic surgical procedures.

Autofluorescence

In the region of cyst formation there is a thinning of the macular pigments that normally attenuate the autofluorescent signal, causing the cysts to appear hyperfluorescent.

Fundus

Cystic prominences form in the macula, frequently having a clover-leaf-like pattern (radially arranged tear drops with their pointed ends toward the fovea). With chronicity cystoid macular edema can cause a tear to form in the inner retinal layers with formation of a macular hole and profound loss of acuity.

Fluorescein Angiography

In the early phase a faint hyperfluorescence is present in the region of the cysts, due to increased transmission of background fluorescence, caused by a reduced density of macular pigment. In the course of the angiogram there is a progressive leakage of fluid from the perifoveal capillaries. Fluorescein collects in the fluid filled spaces, which becomes clearer as the background fluorescence fades. In the late phase of the angiogram the dye filled cavities look like multiple cysts.

◘ **Fig. 5.26a–f.** A 42 year old patient with uveitis and cystoid macular edema in the left eye. Fundoscopically **a** and with infrared imaging **b**, one can see the individual macular cysts. Autofluorescence angiography **c** shows the cysts with a hyperfluorescence due to thinning of the macular pigments. Fluorescein angiography **d–f** shows the gradual filling of the individual cysts with fluorescein. Typical clover-leaf-like hyperfluorescent cysts in the late phase **f**.

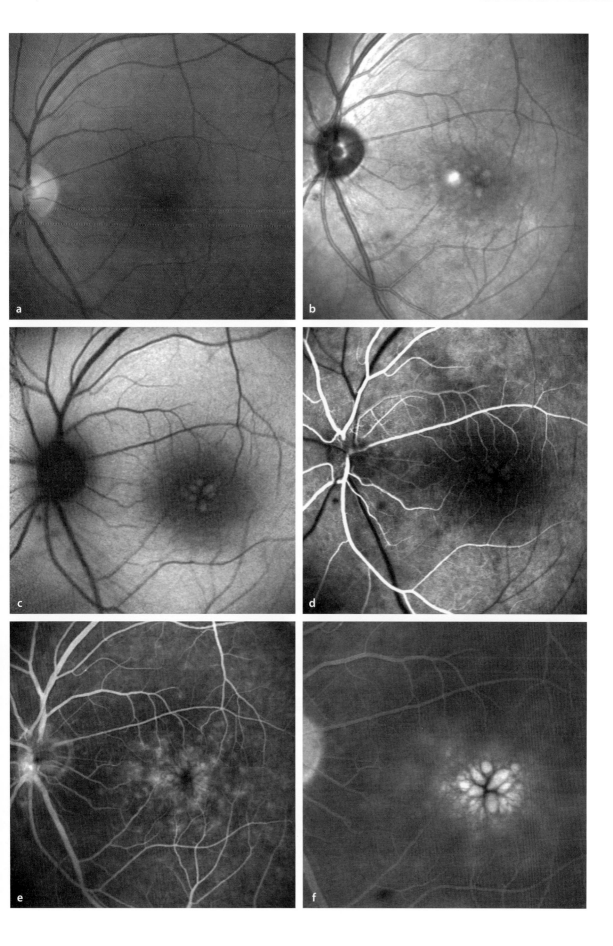

5.3 Hereditary Macular Disorders

5.3.1 Stargardt's Disease

Stargardt's disease is the most common hereditary macular dystrophy. Usually an autosomal recessive trait (mutations in the ABCA4 gene) it is characterized by excessive lipofuscin storage in the RPE cells and a subsequent loss of the RPE cells. The process can remain limited to the macula (Stargardt's disease) and/or affect the periphery (fundus flavimaculatus). Stargardt's disease usually manifests itself in the second decade of life, but can also appear in later decades (late onset, ◘ Fig. 4.6e).

Symptoms
Presents as a loss of acuity and a central visual field defect.

Fundus
The clinical picture of Stargardt's disease can be highly variable. Early in the course of the disease the fundus can still have a normal appearance. Then the foveal reflex fades from view and the fovea acquires a granular and indistinct appearance. Surrounding the fovea there arise a number of concentrically oriented, pale yellow specks at the level of the RPE. This is caused by a marked accumulation of lipofuscin within the RPE cells, which displaces the melanin granules towards the cell borders. Later, an obliquely oval zone of degeneration develops containing fine flecks of RPE destruction. The fovea appears dark and is surrounded by hypo- and hyperpigmented rings (so-called target maculopathy). The central RPE can show many areas of geographic atrophy.

Autofluorescence
In areas where the RPE has been destroyed, autofluorescence is extinguished. An increase in autofluorescence can be found corresponding to areas of lipofuscin deposition in the regions with the pale yellow flecks.

Fluorescein Angiography
Due to the lipofuscin accumulation in the RPE, the background fluorescence of the choroid is blocked or weakened (dark choroid). In areas where the RPE is missing the choroidal fluorescence is unobstructed, a phenomenon referred to as window defects. The RPE defects can be demonstrated much more effectively by angiography than by ophthalmoscopy. The ophthalmoscopically visible pale yellow flecks appear hyperfluorescent during fluorescein angiography.

5.3.2 Fundus Flavimaculatus

The pale yellow flecks at the RPE level, as described above for Stargardt's disease, can also appear without any macular involvement. In this form the disese is called fundus flavimaculatus. It is thought that Stargardt's disease and fundus flavimaculatus are two different phenotypic expressions of the same disease. Both phenotypes can also be found together.

◘ **Fig. 5.27a–f.** A 30 year old patient with Stargardt's disease. **a** Fundoscopy of the right eye shows an obliquely oval central area of degeneration with tiny spots of RPE damage. Within the area of degeneration there is an island of preserved RPE. Surrounding the zone of degeneration one can see scattered white flecks. **b** Autofluorescence imaging shows that within the zone of degeneration the RPE is completely atrophic and there is no longer any visible autofluorescence. The small island of preserved RPE cells is marked by a patch of persistent autofluorescence. Surrounding the zone of degeneration there is a ring of flecks with markedly elevated autofluorescence. These spots correlate with the funduscopically visible white flecks, and reflect the elevated levels of intracellular RPE lipofuscin. **c,d** Fluorescein angiography shows transmitted background choroidal fluorescence in the area of missing RPE cells (a type of window defect). No leakage is apparent. **e,f** The left eye has a similar appearance.

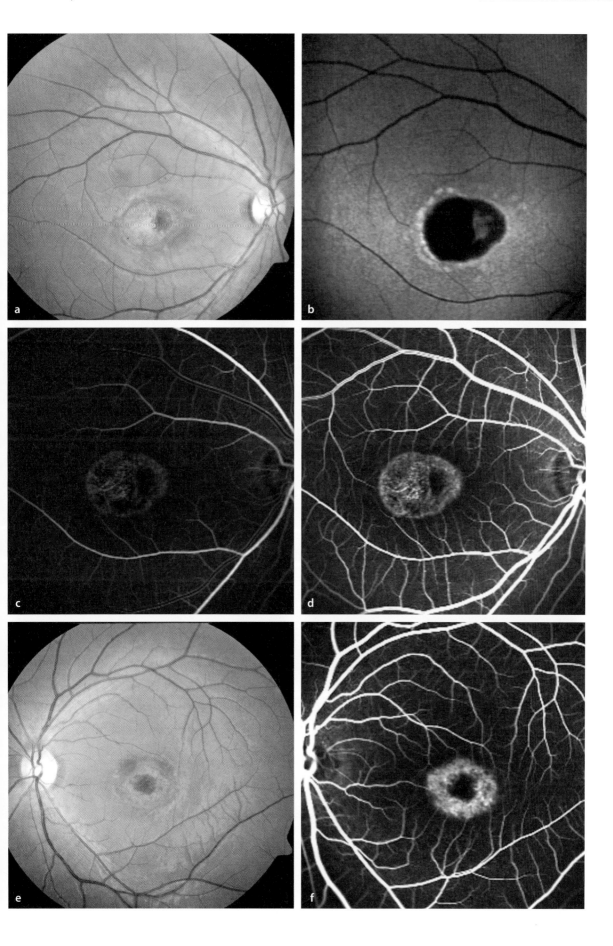

5.3.3 Best's Disease (Vitelliform Macular dystrophy)

Best's disease is an autosomal dominant macular dystrophy with incomplete penetrance, caused by a mutation in the so-called VMD2-gene, expressed in the RPE. This disorder is usually first manifest in the second decade of life, although late presentations have also been described. It affects both eyes and has a course that goes through several stages. Characteristic is a reduced or absent light rise in the electrooculogram (EOG). A complicating factor in some cases is the appearance of choroidal neovascularization with the dystrophic macula.

Fundus

Initially thee is an egg-yolk-like (vitelliform), yellow, disc-shaped change in the macula with a diameter larger than one disc diameter. This is caused by a massive accumulation of lipofuscin in the cells of the RPE. Visual function at this stage is normal. Later on there is destruction of the RPE with increasing release of lipofuscin into the subretinal space. This gives the clinical impression of a destruction and liquefaction of the contents of the macular lesion, accompanied by formation of a »pseudohypopyon«. Later on there is a mixture of yellow material and scar tissue, and in the atrophic stage there is no longer any visible yellow pigment.

Autofluorescence

The disc shaped accumulation of lipofuscin is easily seen, given its strong autofluorescence.

Fluorescein Angiography

Given the unmistakeable ophthalmoscopic appearance of Best's disease and positive EOG findings, a fluorescein angiogram is not necessary. Angiography merely confirms the attenuation of the background fluorescence by lipofuscin. In advanced stages the areas of RPE destruction are visible as window defects, meaning that the background fluorescence is transmitted. A fluorescein angiogram is indicated when there is a suspicion of a CNVM.

◘ Fig. 5.28a–f. a The right eye of a young patient with a highly reflective fundus image and the central vitteliform changes of Best's disease. Visual acuity is 20/20, and EOG shows reduced light rise. **b** Markedly increased autofluorescence in the visibly affected central area. **c** The contralateral eye likewise has a vitelliform lesion, in which additional vessels can be seen. Visual acuity is 20/125 and there is a reduced light rise in the EOG. The vitelliform lesion is surrounded by a region of subretinal fluid and shallow hemorrhages. Its borders are sharply demarcated by distinct retinal surface reflections. **d–f** Fluorescein angiography of the left eye shows attenuation of the background fluorescence by the subretinal blood and exudation. In the area of the vitelliform lesion one can see a secondary CNV membrane, which shows leakage of dye during the course of the angiogram **f**.

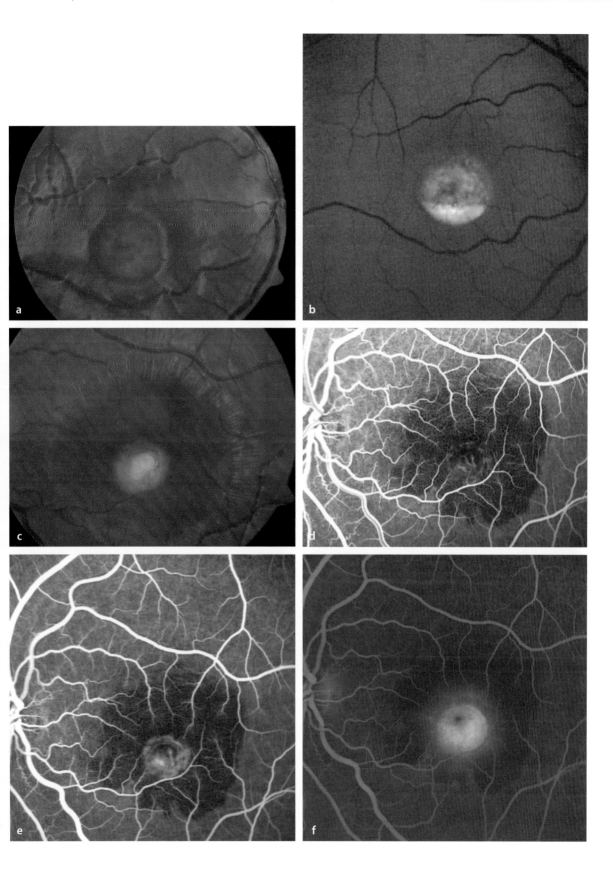

5.3.4 Pattern Dystrophies of the Retinal Pigment Epithelium (RPE)

The pattern dystrophies of the RPE constitute a varied group of maculopathies that all have bilateral, symmetrical, pattern-like changes in the RPE. An autosomal dominant mode of inheritance has been described. Pattern dystrophies are often manifest at mid-life.

Symptoms

Visual acuity is usually normal or minimally reduced. Visual field and ERG tests are both largely unaffected.

Fundus

Fundoscopically there are bilateral pigmented lines arrayed in typical patterns, including among others butterfly shaped RPE dystrophy and reticular RPE dystrophy. Most of these patterns have the pigmented lines arranged in a radial fashion.

Autofluorescence

Pattern dystrophies are more easily seen by autofluorescence than by conventional ophthalmoscopy.

Fluorescein Angiography

The pigmented lines partially block transmission of background fluorescence, making their pattern of changes in the RPE stand out clearly during angiography. Since the pigmented lines are hyperfluorescent on autofluorescence images and hypofluorescent on fluorescein angiographic images, autofluorescence images look somewhat like the negatives of a fluorescein angiographic study.

Fig. 5.29a–e. A 72 year old patient with pattern dystrophy of the RPE. **a** Fundoscopy reveals pigmented lines arrayed in a radial pattern. **b,c** The pigmented lines have a clearly elevated level of autofluorescence. **d,e** Fluorescein angiography: The blockage of background fluorescence by the pigmented lines makes the pattern and extent of the dystrophy clear. There is no leakage of dye.

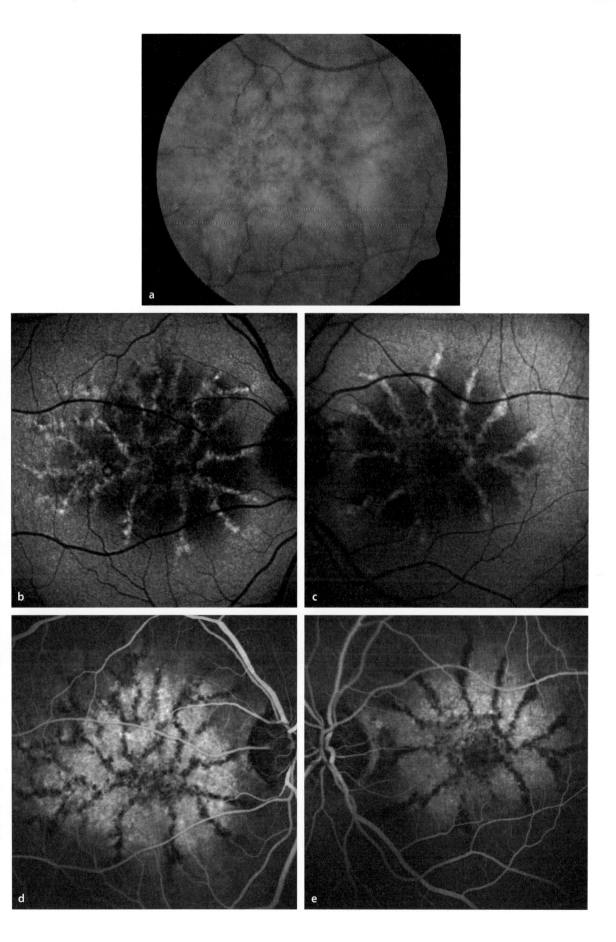

5.3.5 Congenital X-Chromosome Retinoschisis

Congenital retinoschisis is an X-linked, recessively inherited disorder that affects males only, while female carriers show no signs of the trait.

Symptoms

Due to the changes in the central visual field, visual acuity is a reduced to a range between 20/50 and 20/100. Patients are often hyperopic. The ERG has reduced B-wave amplitudes.

Fundus

In the macula there is typically a star-shaped distortion of the inner limiting membrane with intraretinal cysts. The changes are often subtle in appearance. The foveal component can be the only expression of this disorder, but up to 70% of patients also have additional areas of schisis in the inferotemporal retinal periphery. In a few cases these changes can lead to intraretinal and/or vitreal hemorrhages.

Fluorescein Angiography

Fluorescein angiography is not necessary for the diagnosis, but will demonstrate the retinal distortion and intraretinal cysts. Leakage of dye is not found.

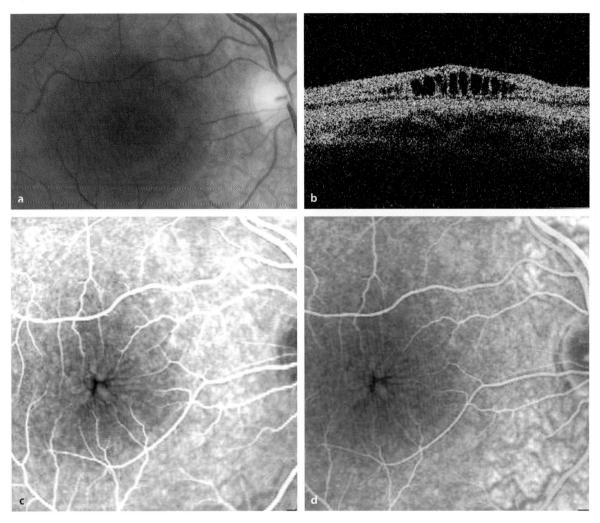

◘ Fig. 5.30a–d. A 20 year old patient with congenital X-linked retinoschisis. Visual acuity is 20/30. **a** Fundoscopy finds delicate, star-shaped distortion of and cyst formation in the macula. **b** OCT imaging demonstrates the intraretinal cysts. **c,d** Fluorescein angiographic images at various times show that there is no leakage of dye, which is exactly the opposite of the findings in cystoid macular edema.

5.4 Adult Vitelliform Macular Degeneration (AVMD)

The term adult vitelliform macular degeneration refers to a genetically heterogeneous group of mid-life disorders in which, yellow lesions appear in the macula. Changes in pigmentation can also be associated with these lesions. In some patients with this disorder a clearly autosomal dominant patter of heredity has been described. The clinical manifestations appear at an older age than do those of Best's disease. The areas of yellow color are generally smaller than a disc diameter and lie at a subretinal level and in the RPE. Despite this, the RPE is not elevated. While AVMD is usually slowly progressive, the yellow pigment can either diminish or increase as the disorder evolves. Finally, the disease transitions into an atrophic end stage. The loss of vision at the beginning of the disorder is relatively mild, and the EOG is normal or only minimally reduced. Complications, such as choroidal neovascularization, seldom develop.

Autofluorescence

Autofluorescence is elevated in the area of the yellow lesions, while pigmented areas block autofluorescence.

Fluorescein Angiography

In the early phase there is blockage of the background fluorescence. In the later course of the study areas of hyperfluorescence can appear in the area of the vitelliform lesion. In contradistinction to an RPE detachment, the late phase does not show homogeneous hyperfluorescence in the area of the lesion.

■ **Fig. 5.31a–f.** A 57 year old patient with adult vitelliform macular degeneration. **a,b** Fundus appearance: yellow lesions, greater in the right eye than in the left. **c,d** Autofluorescence images: the lesions are hyperfluorescent. **e,f** Fluorescein angiography: irregular hyperfluorescence without increase in size in the areas of the lesions with simultaneous partial blockage of the background fluorescence.

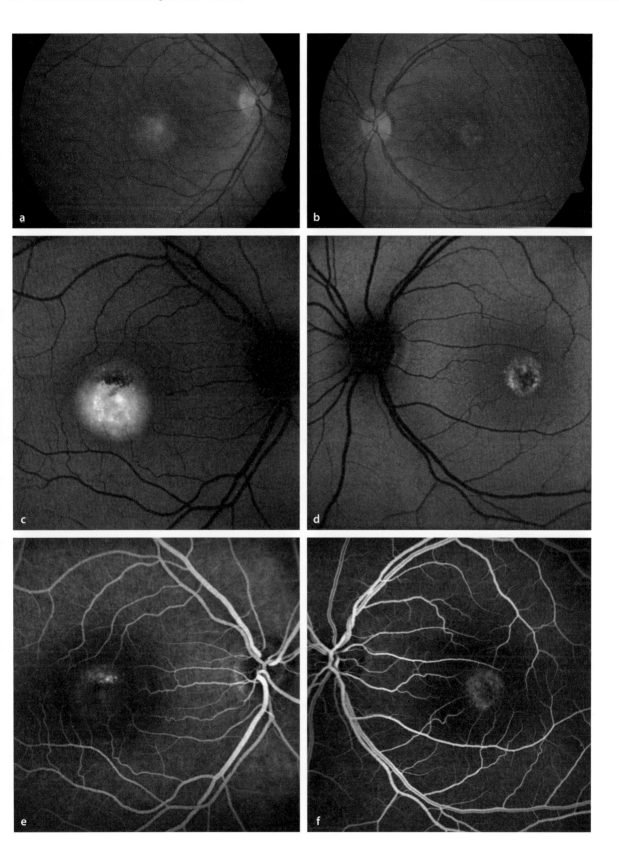

5.5   The Macular Degeneration of Myopia

High myopia develops with excessive growth in the axial length of the eye, which leads to an elongation of the posterior segment. This causes a thinning of all layers of the ocular wall.

Fundus

With thinning of the ocular wall a posterior staphyloma can develop, surrounding the optic disc, or located in other areas of the posterior pole. Thinning of the RPE leads to a generally lighter fundus appearance with zones of RPE atrophy. The juxtapapillary RPE retracts from the optic disc, giving rise to an initially temporal and then later a peripapillary conus. Likewise, and depending on the degree of thinning, breaks can appear in Bruch's membrane, which are funduscopically visible as depigmented, bright lines (so-called »lacquer cracks«). These can be accompanied by subretinal hemorrhages, which later organize and leave behind a pigmented scar (also referred to as Fuchs' fleck). Centers of thinning appear as chorioretinal zones of atrophy in the posterior pole that appear white with transmission of light reflected by the sclera, and which in some cases may still contain large choroidal vessels. With time, these centers can enlarge and/or merge with one another. Choroidal neovascularization can appear at the margins of the lacquer cracks, at the edges of ocular wall ectatic areas, and in other locations. Compared to the CNV associated with AMD, these are relatively small and are as a rule accompanied by small hemorrhages, or smaller serous detachments of the retina. The CNV lesions can be surrounded by a pigmented ring.

Fluorescein Angiography

The breaks in Bruch's membrane are easily visible during fluorescein angiography, due to the transmission of background fluorescence. In the areas of ocular wall ectasias background fluorescence is missing, due to atrophy of the choriocapillaris. Large choroidal vessels that have remained are easily visible. Retinal capillaries and the foveal avascular zone are, as a rule, poorly defined. The most important indication for a fluorescein angiogram is suspicion of a CNV.

◨ **Fig. 5.32a,b.** A 20 year old patient with high myopia. **a** Fundoscopy. There is a peripapillary conus and a linear, extended course of the retinal vessels. Beneath the fovea there is an S-shaped, bright line, a typical »lacquer crack« (*arrow*). **b** Fluorescein angiography demonstrates the hyperfluorescence of the lacquer crack, in the sense of its property as a window defect.

◨ **Fig. 5.33a–d.** A 59 year old patient with high myopia. **a** Fundoscopy reveals a peripapillary conus and an atrophic, chorioretinal region of ocular wall ectasia that reaches to the fovea. **b–d** In the early phase the fluorescein angiogram shows a small, classic CNV right at the margin of an ectatic area (*arrow*). The CNV is hyperfluorescent and is surrounded by a narrow hypofluorescent border. In the late phase there is significant leakage of dye from the CNV.

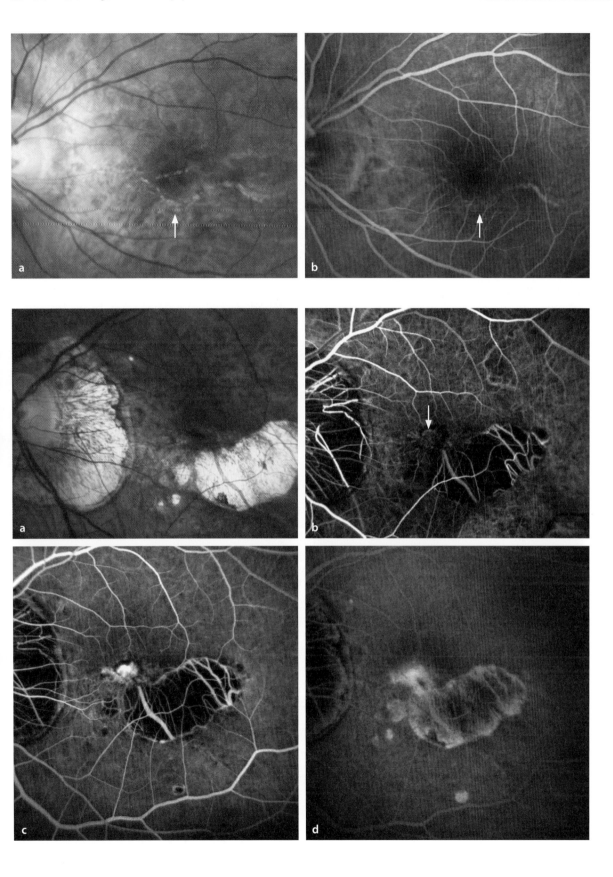

5.6   Angioid Streaks

Angioid streaks are dehiscences in Bruch's membrane that can be isolated findings or can be seen in the context of syndromes, such as pseudoxanthoma elasticum, the Ehlers-Danlos syndrome, Paget's disease, or sickle-cell anemia. The clinical importance of angiod streaks rests primarily on the tendency of CNV membranes to originate at their margins.

Fundus

The changes are called angioid streaks, since with the break in Bruch's membrane the dark red color of the choroidal vessels can be seen, giving the break a vessel-like appearance. The streaks extend from the peripapillary region and branch out peripherally as they taper in width. Often the breaks form a ring that surrounds the optic disc. Pseudoxanthoma elasticum can also be associated with a so-called »peau d'orange« appearance, a degenerative process in Bruch's membrane that gives the fundus a coarse granular appearance, especially in the region temporal to the macula.

Fluorescein Angiography

Atrophy of the RPE can develop in areas of angioid streaks. Consequently, the background fluorescence is transmitted and the streaks appear as hyperfluorescent lines. The hyperfluorescence corresponds to the extent of RPE atrophy, but not of the angioid streaks. Ophthalmoscopically visible angioid streaks, depending on circumstances, cannot be detected by fluorescein angiography. Fluorescein angiographic images of the »peau d'orange« areas are generally unremarkable.

ICG Angiography

During the early phase of an ICG angiogram the angioid streaks are not apparent. In the late phase of the study angioid streaks appear hyperfluorescent and are (in comparison to the ophthalmoscopic and fluorescein angiographic findings) clearly defined. In some cases the streaks are detectable only by ICG angiography. This may be due to binding of the ICG to components within the streaks, such as the debris left by degenerated elastin. Corresponding to the funduscopically visible areas of »peau d'orange«, plaque shaped areas of hyperfluorescence appear in the late phase, indicating that the areas of degeneration also have a higher affinity for free ICG.

■ **Fig. 5.34a–f. a** A 39 year old patient with pseudoxanthoma elasticum (PXE) has a central area of acute hemorrhage in the presence of angioid streaks. **b** Fluorescein angiography shows the peripapillary angioid streaks as hyperfluorescent lines. At the temporal border of the hemorrhage one can see a secondary CNV close to an angioid streak. **c** Peripapillary angioid streaks in a 20 year old patient with PXE. **d** 30 minutes following an ICG injekction, angiod streaks – some oriented radial, others parallel to the disc – are seen as hyperfluorescent lines. **e** Angioid streaks are also easy to see in fundus autofluorescence images. **f** Late phase ICG image in a patient with angioid streaks and PXE. In addition to the hyperfluorescent angioid streaks there are temporal (right side of image) prominent, partially confluent plaque-like foci of hyperfluorescence that correlate with the »peau d'orange« fundus appearance.

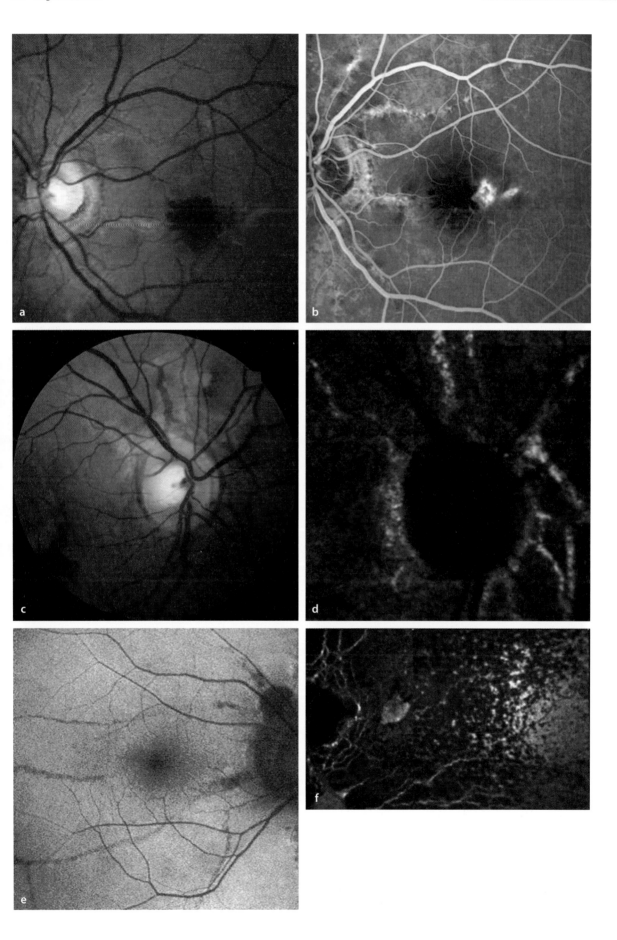

5.7   Central Serous Chorioretinopathy (CSC)

(Various synonyms: »Retinopathy, central serous« (RSC), »idiopathic central serous chorioretinopathy« (ICSC), and »idiopathic chorioretinopathy, central serous« (ICCS))

CSC is a circumscribed elevation of the neuroretina (and often the RPE as well), located in the posterior pole, and caused by a disturbance of the blood-retinal barrier. It is usually unilateral. The cause of CSC is unknown, although it often develops in connection with corticosteroid therapy or during a pregnancy. It occurs most often in patients aged 20 to 50 years, and men are more frequently affected than women.

Symptoms

Poor visual acuity, relative central scotoma, blurred vision, disturbances of color perception, and poor dark adaptation.

Fundus

There is a disc-shaped, circumscribed elevation of the neuroretina. The retinal vessels and the optic disc are unaffected.

Fluorescein Angiography

In the early phase there is an attenuation of choroidal fluorescence by subretinal fluid. The next event is leakage of fluorescein into the subretinal cystic space(s) that overlie(s) sites of pathological change in the RPE. In 90% of patients there is only one such source of leakage. Further into the study there is a generally circular spread of the initially punctuate hyperfluorescence. In 25% of patients there is a so-called »smoke stack« configuration (also called an umbrella sign): one can see that the dye inside the subretinal cyst first climbs upward to collect in the superior portions of the cyst. The differential diagnosis should include idiopathic choroidal neovascularization, which must be ruled out.

◨ Fig. 5.35a,b. A 43 year old patient with acute onset of metamorphopsia. **a** Fundoscopy reveals a well demarcated subretinal area of fluid accumulation that includes the fovea. **b** Fluorescein angiography shows an area of subretinal fluid that partially blocks the background fluorescence. Inside this area is a point source of dye leakage.

◨ Fig. 5.36a–d. A 42 year old patient with metamorphopsia in the left eye, caused by central serous chorioretinopathy (CSC). **a–d** fluorescein angiography: there is a central shadowing of the background fluorescence due to an accumulation of subretinal fluid. Nasal and inferior to the macula there is a point source of dye leakage, which rises inside the cystic space (smoke stack phenomenon), and then gradually fills the cystic space to show its full extent.

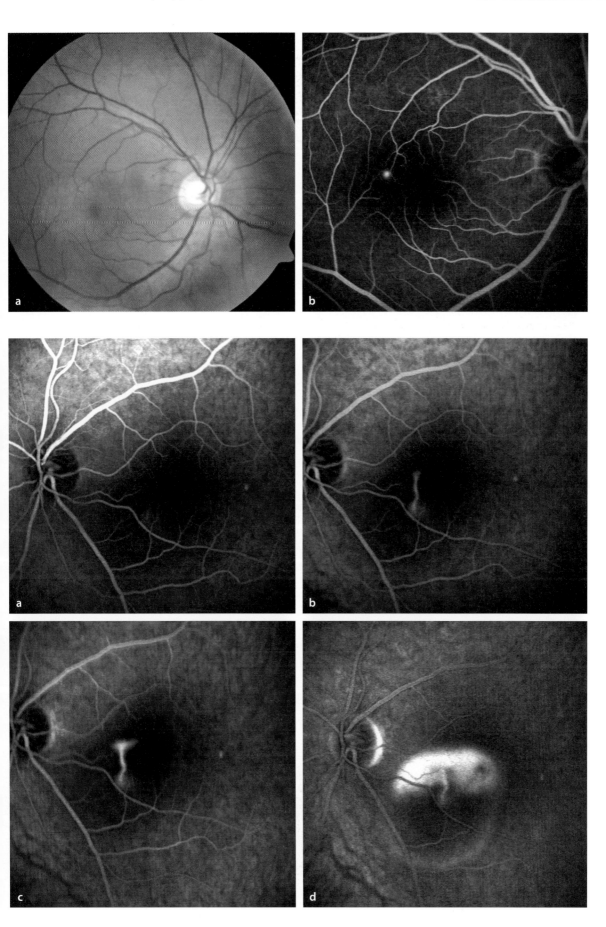

5.8   Chronic Idiopathic Central Serous Chorioretinopathy (CICSC)

(Synonym: »diffuse retinal pigment epitheliopathy«)

Fundus

In contrast with the description above of central serous chorioretinopathy having a solitary source of dye leakage, CICSC presents with one or more zones of diffuse RPE changes, for which reason the disorder is also called diffuse pigment epitheliopathy. In the area of RPE changes there are chronic relapsing areas of leakage with corresponding visual impairment, chiefly reduced acuity and metamorphopsia.

Fluorescein Angiography

In the regions of pathological RPE zones there are irregular patterns of fluorescence with juxtaposed flecks of hyper- and hypo-fluorescence. In the late phase there is a slow, diffuse escape of fluorescein from these areas – a subtle form of leakage.

ICG Angiography

Corresponding to the pathological changes seen during fluorescein angiography, increased fluorescence appears in the same locations during ICG angiograms. The ICG hyperfluorescence spreads out and then gradually fades. Similar changes can also be found in the contralateral eye.

Fig. 5.37a–f. A 46 year old patient with chronic idiopathic central serous chorioretinopathy. **a** Fundoscopy of the right eye shows pathological areas of RPE nasal and inferonasal to the fovea. **b–d** Fluorescein angiography shows that affected areas develop irregular, patchy areas of hyperfluorescence with development of limited dye leakage in the late phase **d**. **e–f** ICG angiography with attention to areas of RPE pathology shows a circumscribed hyperfluorescence that then fades during the later course of the study **f**.

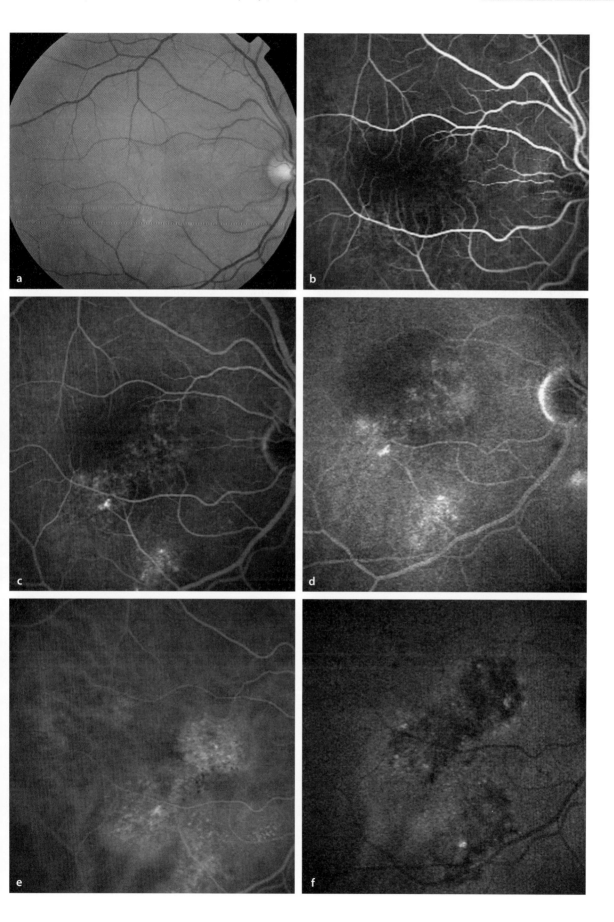

5.9   Idiopathic Juxtafoveal Teleangiectasias

This disorder presents with irregular, dilated ectasias of retinal capillaries, primarily temporal to the fovea. The cause is unknown. The juxtafoveal teleangiectasias lead to chronic macular edema, eventually developing an accumulation of hard exudates. In advanced stages tissue atrophy and/or areas of choroidal neovascularization develop (in Type 2). This disorder has been classified as having two types:

Type 1 (aneurysmal telangiectasias): the aneurysmal changes in retinal vessels are funduscopically visible. This is usually a monocular presentation, affecting men more frequently, usually in mid-life.

Type 2 (perifoveal telangiectasias): The altered sections of vessels are not funduscopically visible, there is instead just a gray discoloration of the perifoveal retinal tissues. There is no sex preference. It appears in patients between 50 and 60 years old.

Fundus

Depending on the type of disorder, one can see a subtle gray discoloration of the perifoveal retina, macular edema, hard exudates and/or visible telangiectasias of vessel segments, particularly temporal to the fovea. With the perifoveal graying of the retina and additional foveal atrophy the funduscopic appearance can resemble that of a lamellar macular hole.

Fluorescein Angiography

Fluorescein angiography demonstrates ectatic segments of retinal blood vessels, particularly in the area temporal to the fovea. During the course of the study one can see leakage in this area.

◻ **Fig. 5.38a–f.** A 50 year old patient with idiopathic juxtafoveal telangiectasias (Type 2). Acuity 20/50 in the right eye, and 20/60 in the left. **a** Fundoscopy demonstrates a perifoveal area of gray discoloration caused by the macular edema. Ectatic segments of the blood vessels are barely visible. **b–d** Fluorescein angiography shows temporal to the fovea a number of ectatic capillaries that are leaking dye **d. e,f** Identical findings are seen in the contralateral eye.

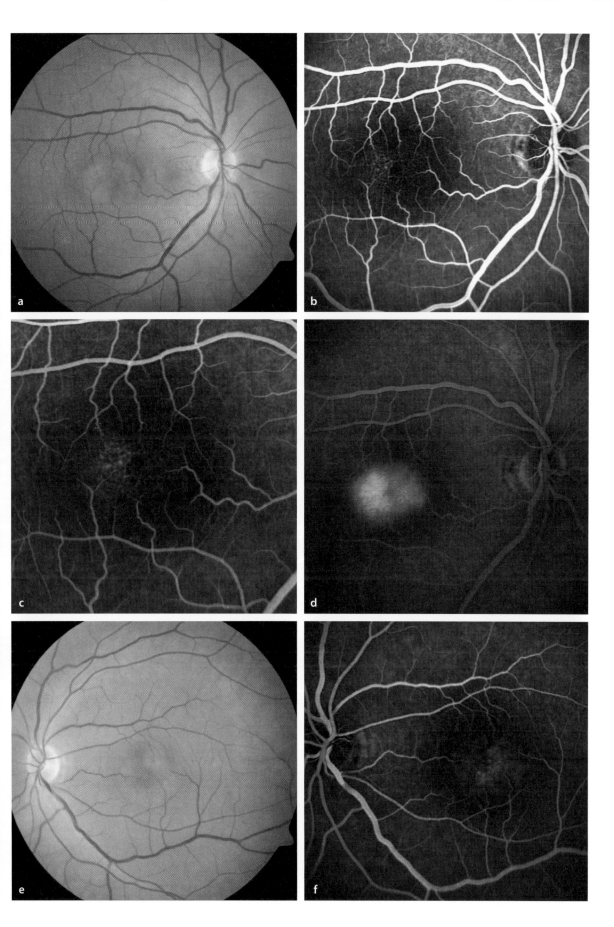

5.10   Epiretinal Gliosis

Central epiretinal membranes can develop in the posterior pole of an eye, caused by a number of pathological entities. They can be idiopathic, caused by retinal vascular disorders (e.g. occlusions of retinal veins, and/or diabetic retinopathy), associated with inflammatory disease (e.g. uveitis), following development of retinal breaks, or after vitreoretinal surgery.

Fundus

Wrinkling of the internal limiting membrane is best seen in red free fundus images. There are vessel segments with corkscrew shapes. Fibrotic epiretinal membranes appear in advanced stages of the process. In some cases a secondary form of cystoid macular edema develops.

Fluorescein Angiography

Epiretinal membranes are best seen in infrared fundus images, while fluorescein angiography is particularly effective in disclosing the extent of vessel distortion and the associated leakage of dye.

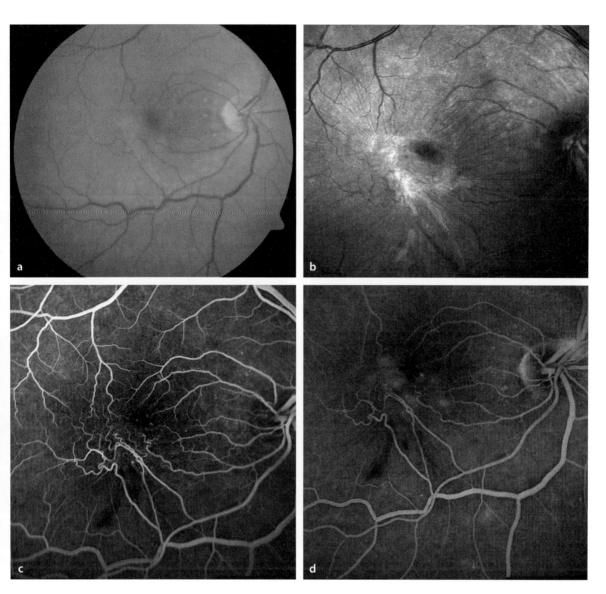

☐ **Fig. 5.39a–d.** A 69 year old patient with progressive metamorphopsia in the right eye. **a** Fundoscopy shows a gray epiretinal membrane inferotemporal to the fovea and a sinuous course of retinal blood vessels in the same region. **b** Infrared images reveal retinal surface details particularly well. Note that the epiretinal membrane has caused wrinkling of the internal limiting membrane and traction of the affected retinal area towards the temporal vascular arcade. **c,d** Fluorescein angiography shows the tortuous course of the affected blood vessels, and demonstrates the associated leakage of dye.

5.11 Macular Holes

The term »macular hole« is most commonly used in reference to an »idiopathic macular hole«, which is an age related disorder found most commonly in older patients. The prevalence is 33/10,000 in patients over 55 years old. Processes at the interface between retina and vitreous result in the development through several stages of a penetrating, central retinal hole.

Autofluorescence / Fluorescein Angiography

Ordinarily, the macular pigment shadows the autofluorescence of the retinal pigment epithelium in the foveal and perifoveal zones, so that autofluorescence images of the retina show a central area of darkness. With formation of a macular hole the macular pigment is missing in the region of the hole, causing a window defect that transmits the autofluorescence of the RPE. For the same reason, a macular hole will appear hyperfluorescent during a fluorescein angiogram of the central retina. As a rule, fluorescein angiography is unnecessary in the diagnosis of a macular hole.

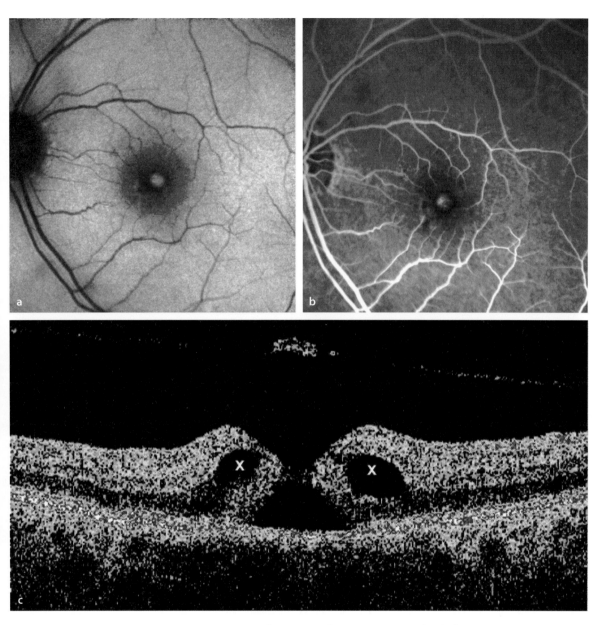

Fig. 5.40a–c. Macular hole, stage 3. **a** Autofluorescence image. In the central macula where the retina is missing, the RPE autofluorescence shines brightly. **b** Fluorescein angiography with an hyperfluorescent macular hole (same patient). **c** Corresponding OCT findings with cystic changes in the retina (x) in the elevated margins surrounding the retinal hole.

5.12   Chloroquine Maculopathy

Long term intake of chloroquine in the treatment of rheumatoid diseases can produce characteristic ocular side effects. A maculopathy develops with optic atrophy, deficits in accommodation, and deposition of pigment in the corneal epithelium (cornea verticillata).

Fundus

Granular, ring-shaped changes in the pigment epithelium of the macula produces a typical picture of a bull's eye maculopathy. As a rule, the maculopathy develops in both eyes.

Autofluorescence / Fluorescein Angiography

The pattern of a bull's eye maculopathy is also found in autofluorescence images with ring shaped zones of alternating elevation and reduction of autofluorescence. Fluorescein angiography is not necessary for the diagnosis.

◨ **Fig. 5.41a–f.** A 60 year old patient with a 17 year history of chloroquine intake for the treatment of systemic lupus erythematosus (cumulative dose of circa 600 g). **a,b** Bilateral bull's eye maculopathy. **c,d** Autofluorescence images show ring-shaped, concentric zones of elevated and depressed auto-fluorescence corresponding to the bull's eye pattern. **e** Central scotoma defined by static perimetry of the central 30 degrees of the visual field. **f** Cornea verticillata (pigmented corneal epithelial deposits) following chloroquine use.

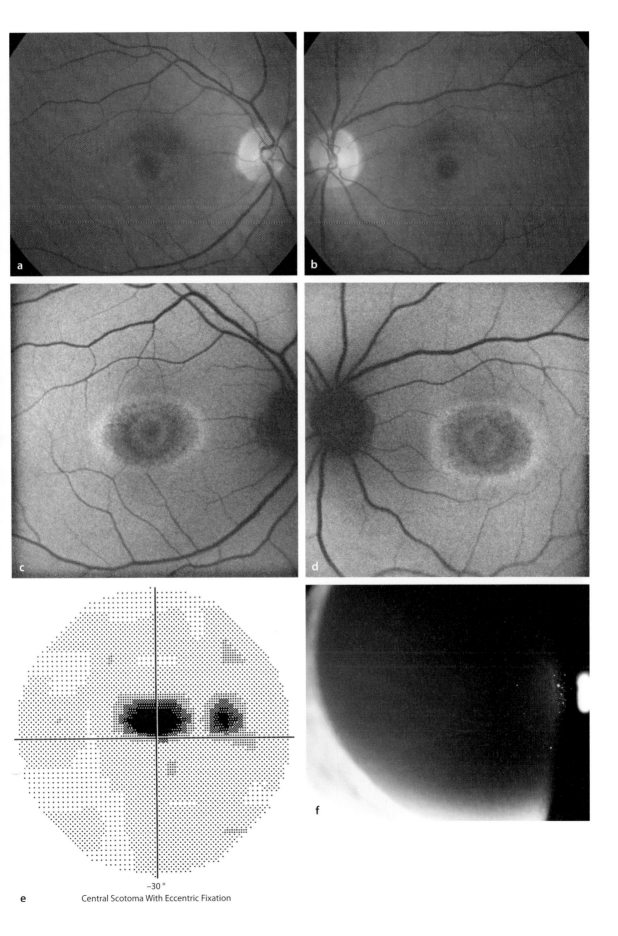

e   Central Scotoma With Eccentric Fixation

−30°

Retinal Vascular Disease

6.1   Diabetic Retinopathy

6.1.1   Nonproliferative Diabetic Retinopathy

Diabetic retinopathy begins with damage to the pericytes and endothelial cells and a thickening of vascular basal lamina. The microangiopathy affects the retina in particular by damaging the precapillary arterioles, capillaries and venules.

Fundus

Depending on the severity of the retinopathy, there are microaneurysms, small retinal hemorrhages, hard exudates, cotton wool spots, macular edema and variations in the caliber of retina venules (so-called »string of pearls«).

Fluorescein Angiography

During fluorescein angiography, **microaneurysms** appear as small, hyperfluorescent dots. Due to structural alterations in the walls of microaneurysms, fluorescein escapes during the course of the study to stain the retinal tissue. Since the fluorescein is almost entirely bound to serum albumin, chronic leakage of dye causes an accumulation of proteinaceous **hard exudates** in the retinal tissue. Such leakage sites can be found at the center of ring shaped accumulations of hard exudates (circinate figures). Fluorescein angiographic studies of these sites usually show a larger number of microaneurysms than can be seen ophthalmoscopically. Microaneurysms can thrombose and atrophy, and are then no longer

angiographically demonstrable. Areas with **hard exudates** and **hemorrhages** block the background fluorescence. Only by angiography is it possible to differentiate clearly between microaneurysms and small hemorrhages. Depending on the severity of diabetic retinopathy, there may be macular edema, which can appear as if it were made up of several cysts, hence the term **cystoid macular edema** (CME). Retinal capillary occlusions lead to areas of non-perfusion that appear hypofluorescent. Vessels that border these areas of non-perfusion frequently show signs of increased permeability. During angiography, those vessels that border areas of capillary non-perfusion frequently leak dye, causing them to become indistinct. Retinal capillaries located adjacent to areas of non-perfusion can become widely enlarged and sinuous, a fundus abnormality that is clinically described as **intraretinal microvascular anomalies (IRMA)**. These can be either dilated segments of pre-existing capillaries, or newly formed elements of intraretinal neovascularization. Loss of perifoveal capillaries can cause an angiographically visible enlargement of the foveal avascular zone. The basis for this tendency is unclear, but these capillaries appear to be particularly sensitive to diabetic damage. Enlargement of the foveal avascular zone often appears early on in the course of the disease with an abnormal dilation of the remaining perifoveal capillaries (in the sense of a compensatory phenomenon). This causes the capillary bed to be more clearly visible during angiography. Enlargement of the avascular zone can result in a distinct reduction in visual function.

Fig. 6.1a–e. A 60 year old patient with diabetic retinopathy. **a** Fundoscopy reveals numerous point-like and blotchy hemorrhages, as well as hard exudates, in the posterior pole. **b–d** Fluorescein angiography shows numerous point-like dots of hyperfluorescence (microaneurysms) that become clearer during the course of the study **c,** causing diffuse macular edema **d. e** Between the retinal vessels are hypofluorescent, non-perfused areas of retina. Capillaries located adjacent to these areas of ischemia are dilated.
f A 50 year old patient with a clearly enlarged foveal avascular zone with the ischemic macular edema of diabetic retinopathy.

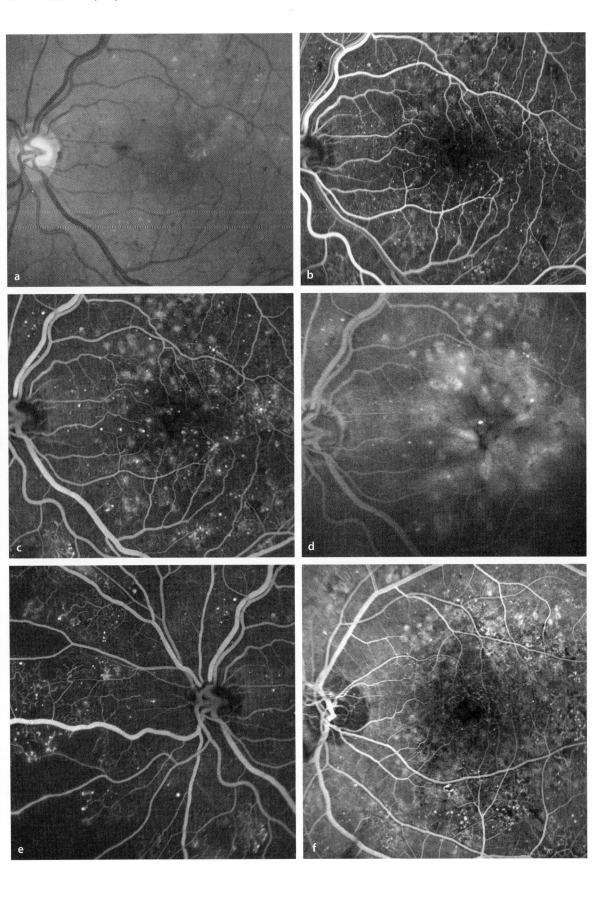

6.1.2 Proliferative Diabetic Retinopathy

In proliferative diabetic retinopathy there is an ischemia-induced production of vascular growth factors (including VEGF, among others) with formation of new vessels. These areas of neovascularization grow (in contrast to the above-mentioned intraretinal microvascular anomalies) through the internal limiting membrane and onto the retinal surface, or arise in other structures like the optic disc, the iris, or the anterior chamber angle.

Fundus

While neovascularization of the anterior chamber angle, iris, and optic disc is usually easy to see, smaller neovascular growths can escape detection during funduscopic examinations, and these are commonly first discovered during fluorescein angiography. Neovascularization often arises close to the margins of retinal areas showing capillary occlusion.

Fluorescein Angiography

Unlike normal retinal vessels, neovascular vessels have fenestrated walls that leak the fluorescent dye. The leakage is initially invisible during the arterial phase of the study, but increases steadily thereafter. When the leakage is very pronounced, the neovascular pattern in the late phase has the appearance of a negative image, i.e. the vessels appear as dark lines against a bright background.

Fig. 6.2a–f. Proliferative diabetic retinopathy. **a** Severe neovascularization of the optic disc. **b** Fluorescein angiography clearly demonstrates leakage of dye from the vessels invading the vitreous body. Through the fluorescent glow of the escaped dye one can see the capillary neovascular segments as tiny, dark lines. **c,d** Peripheral retinal neovascularization, which can be seen more easily by angiography than by funduscopy. **e,f** Retrohyaloid hemorrhage inferior to the macula with blockage of background fluorescence. Peripheral to the hemorrhage are areas of neovascularization reaching into the vitreous body.

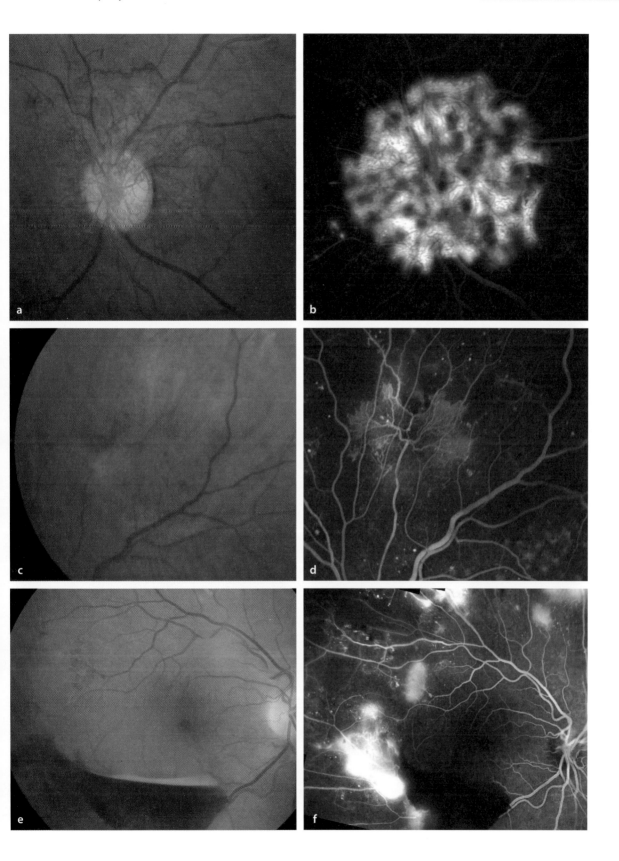

6.2 Hypertensive Retinopathy

Chronic arterial hypertension can lead to a narrowing of the retinal arterioles and a decrease in the perfusion of areas within the retinal capillary bed. Typically, the results of the vascular changes lead to formation of so-called crossing signs at the intersection of retinal arterioles and venules. Depending on the severity of the hypertension, one can also find hypertensive changes in the choroidal vessels.

Fundus

The decreased capillary perfusion can lead to circumscribed areas of ischemia in the nerve fiber layer, which are seen ophthalmoscopically as soft white exudates (»cotton wool spots«). The hypertensive damage can also damage the inner blood-retinal barrier, resulting in escape of serous proteins (seen as hard exudates) and blood into the extravascular retinal tissue.

Fluorescein Angiography

In the areas of cotton wool spots there is a blockage of the fluorescence phenomena, i.e. hypofluorescence. Poorly perfused retinal areas also appear hypofluorescent. Hypertensive damage in the choroid is seen as a delayed filling of choroidal vessels and/or segmental filling of the choroid.

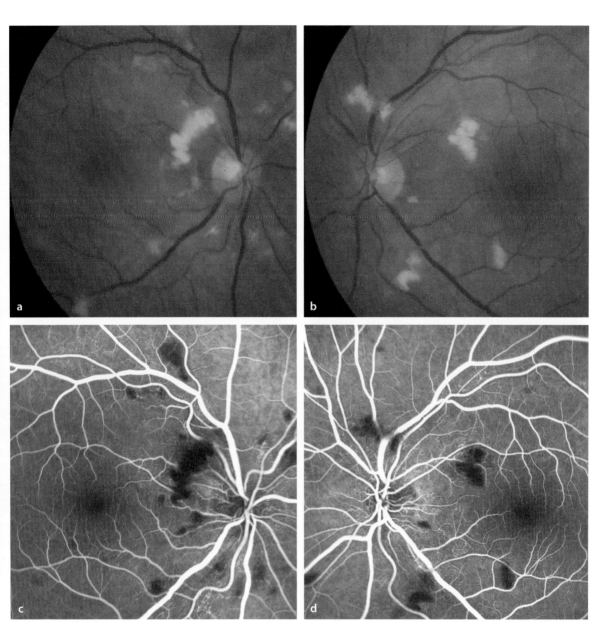

◘ Fig. 6.3a–d. A 52 year old patient presents with bilateral loss of vision. **a,b** Fundoscopy finds multiple cotton-wool spots. **c,d** These spots are localized regions of ischemia in the nerve fiber layer of the retina, and they produce a blockage of background fluorescence. The patient had no past history of hypertension. Systolic blood pressure was 220 mmHg.

6.3   Retinal Arterial Occlusions

6.3.1   Occlusion of the Central Retinal Artery

Occlusion of the central retinal artery occurs most commonly at or near the lamina cribrosa, and is usually caused by thrombosis, embolism, or vasculitis.

Fundus

Occlusion of the central retinal artery produces edema in the inner layers of the retina with loss of transparency in the retinal tissue. Since loss of transparency does not involve the fovea, as it does the surrounding region of the retina, the red color of the choroid is visible at the fovea and the surrounding retina appears white and opaque. This is the cause of the »cherry red spot«. If there is a cilioretinal artery (found in 30% of normal eyes). The area supplied by the cilioretinal artery is not affected by infarction of other retinal areas, since the cilioretinal artery receives its blood supply from the choroidal circulation. This can spare all or part of the papillomacular bundle, preserving both the retina's appearance and the eye's visual acuity. In some cases emboli can be identified in the peripheral retinal arterioles.

Fluorescein Angiography

The funduscopic findings are diagnostic, meaning that angiography is usually not necessary. It shows delayed filling of the arterial vascular tree. After a central retinal artery occlusion, re-canalization and reperfusion of the occluded segments of arterioles is common. The retinal vessels remain, but are very narrow, since the oxygen requirement of the atrophic retina is low. Complete closure is very uncommon. There is almost always some degree of retained perfusion.

6.3.2   Branch Retinal Artery Occlusion

Closure of a branch retinal artery is usually embolic. The occlusion is often incomplete, so that some degree of perfusion persists.

Fundus

The infarcted areas of retina are discolored white, due to the ischemic retinal edema. The blood columns in the occluded vessels appear thread-like and segmented. Sometimes an embolus can be prominently visible at the site of occlusion.

Autofluorescence

The retinal edema blocks autofluorescence. Embolic material can also show autofluorescence.

Fluorescein Angiography

Where the infarcted retina is edematous, the background fluorescence is blocked. The affected retinal vessels fill only very slowly. In some cases, there is even some retrograde filling of an occluded arteriole. At the site of the intravascular embolus, hypofluorescent sparing can be striking.

◨ **Fig. 6.4a–f.** A 58 year old patient with occlusion of the inferotemporal branch of the central retinal artery in the left eye. **a** Fundoscopy shows a white embolus close to the optic disc. There is a broad area of retinal edema in the region supplied by the occluded artery. **b** Autofluorescent imaging: The embolus shows autofluorescence. The edematous area of retina blocks the normal background auto-fluorescence. **c–f** Fluorescein angiography: initially there is no filling of the affected vessels. Due to the reduced arterial blood flow, the inferotemporal vein also shows delayed filling. Gradually, there is segmental filling of the inferotemporal artery, which is largely from retrograde flow, while at the site of occlusion only a tiny bit of fluorescein gets through.

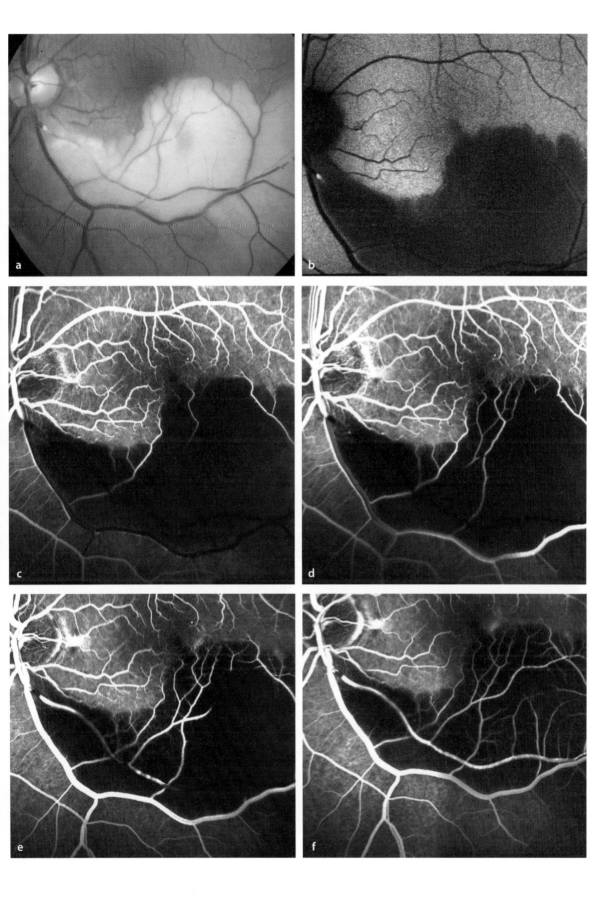

6.4   Retinal Vein Occlusions

Retinal venous occlusions occur in variable locations and with differing extents. Depending on the site of the occlusion, one can differentiate central retinal vein occlusions (CRVO), hemiretinal vein occlusions (HRVO), tributary vein occlusions (TVO), and macular tributary vein occlusions.

6.4.1   Central Retinal Vein Occlusion (CRVO)

In central retinal vein occlusions the site of obstruction to blood flow lies at the level of the lamina cribrosa. Depending on the severity of the occlusion, the clinical manifestations of a CRVO are highly variable. In the past classification by degree of severity in CRVO was the topic of numerous and in part controversial publications. Today, the classification originally used by the Central Vein Occlusion Study Group (CVOSG), beginning in the early 1990's, has found the greatest acceptance. The most important parameter for classifying vein occlusion is the degree of retinal ischemia. A non-ischemic CRVO is usually an incomplete occlusion of the central retinal vein. Perfusion of blood and its oxygen content is still sufficient to avoid development of ischemic retinopathy with its secondary neovascularization. On the other hand a CRVO is ischemic if rubeosis of the iris or retinal neovascularization are already present, or if fluorescein angiography finds that there are 10 or more disc areas of retinal ischemia, which is regarded as a very high risk for development of neovascularization. Because flat retinal hemorrhages block the background hyperfluorescence, they make classification of CRVO's impossible. The CVOSG found that 83% of patients having flat retinal hemorrhages in a setting of CRVO had to be classified as ischemic, based on their findings in later stages of the angiographic studies. This means that the presence of flat retinal hemorrhages is an indication of the presence of or an impending conversion to an ischemic CRVO.

Fundus

The spectrum ranges from a subtle intraluminal elevation of pressure in the central retinal vein with a few isolated hemorrhages, to widespread, confluent areas of flat retinal hemorrhage with ischemic complications, including neovascular glaucoma.

Fluorescein Angiography

Fluorescein angiography shows delayed venous filling and a disturbance of the inner blood-retinal barrier, indicated by increasing leakage of dye during the course of the study. In regions of retinal ischemia (so-called »areas of capillary non-perfusion«) there is hypofluorescence. By the criteria of the CVOSG, differentiation of perfused versus ischemic CRVO is possible by angiography, as long as retinal hemorrhages are not widespread and do not block the fluorescence phenomena. An avascular region of more than 10 times the area of one optic disc carries a high risk for development of neovascularization, while an area of capillary non-perfusion of less than 5 times one disc area has a very low risk of neovascularization. Fluorescein angiography makes an important contribution when differentiating between neovascular and optocilliary shunt vessels. The latter type refers to preformed shunt vessels between the retinal and choroidal circulation. In the event of a central retinal vein occlusion, and within 2 to 3 months, these vessels can expand to create an alternative conduit that shunts blood from the retinal venous system into the choroid, where the blood escapes the eye through the vortex veins. These shunt vessels are visible on the surface of the optic disc and are very difficult to differentiate from papillary neovascularization, based on their ophthalmoscopic appearance. Fluorescein angiography identifies neovascular vessels (in contradistinction to shunt vessels) by their leakage of the angiographic dye. Leakage is the result of high permeability in the walls of the newly formed vessels that permits relatively small molecular weight substances like fluorescein molecules to pass freely.

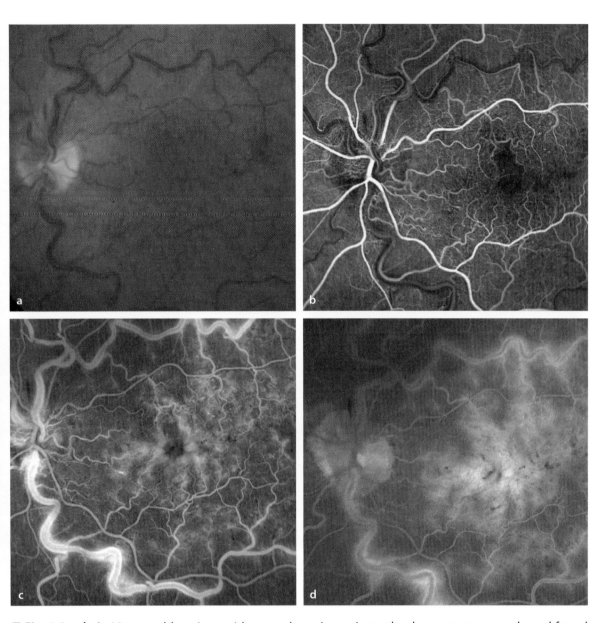

■ **Fig. 6.5a–d.** A 66 year old patient with central retinal vein occlusion in the left eye with visual acuity reduced to 20/100. **a** Fundoscopy shows plainly engorged and sinuous central veins and numerous small intraretinal hemorrhages. **b–d** Fluorescein angiography demonstrates an enlarged foveal avascular zone. Filling of the retinal veins is clearly delayed. In the later course of the angiogram there is a pronounced accumulation of cystoid macular edema.

◼ **Fig. 6.6a,b.** A 70 year old patient with a central retinal vein occlusion in the right eye. **a** The central retinal vein is engorged and sinuous. There are both streaks of hemorrhage in the nerve fiber layer and deeper intraretinal hemorrhages. The arterial vascular tree is reduced in caliber, and there are portions of the arterioles in which white lines are seen in place of the arteries. Neovascularization is not visible. **b** Fluorescein angiography shows the considerable extent of the retinal ischemia: large retinal areas show no perfusion of blood. These areas of capillary non-perfusion are surrounded by enlarge vessels with tortuous shapes, which are preformed shunt vessels and not neovascular growths.

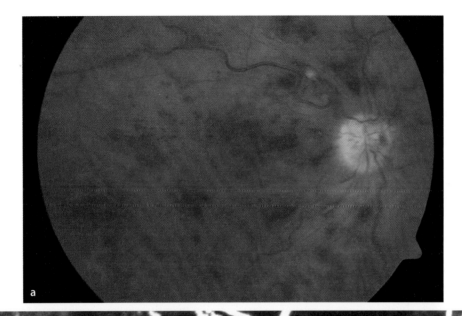

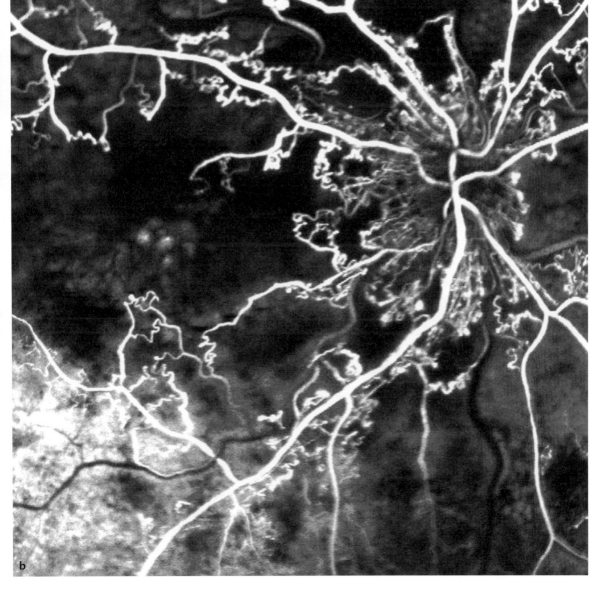

6.4.2 Tributary Retinal Vein Occlusion

Tributary retinal vein occlusions can be classified as primary tributary vein occlusions and macular tributary vein occlusions. With primary tributary vein occlusions an area of more than 10 times the optic disc area can be affected. Analogous to the criteria of the CVOSG for ischemic and non-ischemic central retinal vein occlusions, one can classify tributary vein occlusions as either ischemic or non-ischemic.

Fundus

Tributary retinal vein occlusions always appear at arteriovenous crossing points. The site of occlusion is almost always where a retinal artery crosses over a vein. This type of crossing is found most frequently in the superotemporal quadrant of the retina. Correspondingly, the region drained by the superotemporal tributary retinal vein is most frequently affected by tributary retinal vein occlusions.

Fluorescein Angiography

More frequently than central retinal vein occlusions (CRVO), tributary retinal vein occlusions (TRVO) show widespread areas of capillary nonperfusion that are demonstrable by fluorescein angiography. At the margins of these areas, one frequently finds enlarged collateral vessels. These can suffer damage to their wall structure by the hypoxia, increasing their permeability and causing a mild degree dye leakage that surrounds the collateral vessels. Neovascularization, on the other hand, leads to a much more severe form of dye leakage. For persistent macular edema in the setting of a TRVO, laser grid photocoagulation can be a useful option. This must be preceded by a fluorescein angiogram to demonstrate a largely intact perifoveal capillary net. Such angiograms, however, can be done only when there has been sufficient resorption of the retinal hemorrhages.

Fig. 6.7a–d. A 68 year old patient with an old occlusion of the superotemporal retinal vein. **a** Fundoscopy reveals the site of the occlusion within one disc diameter of the superotemporal disc margin. The accompanying artery crosses over the vein at this point. The affected vessel shows secondary sheathing by a local proliferation of glial cells. In addition one can see small hemorrhages, hard exudates and dilated vessel segments in the area drained by the occluded vein. **b–d** Fluorescein angiography: The superotemporal vein fills very slowly. There are areas of capillary nonperfusion and dilated segments of preformed arteriovenous shunt vessels. Easily seen are the numerous dilated collateral vessels that cross the horizontal meridian, joining the superotemporal quadrant with the inferotemporal quadrant. In the late phase (**d**) there is a limited degree of leakage from the shunt vessels, caused by hypoxic damage to their wall structure.

Fig. 6.8a,b. A 69 year old patient with a macular tributary vein occlusion in the right eye. the affected area of fundus is smaller than 5 disc areas, for which reason the risk of ischemic complications is low. **a,b** Fluorescein angiography: In the affected area there are no identifiable capillaries. The larger vessels crossing the ischemic area have suffered hypoxic damage to their walls, producing some leakage of dye (**b**) in the late phase of the study.

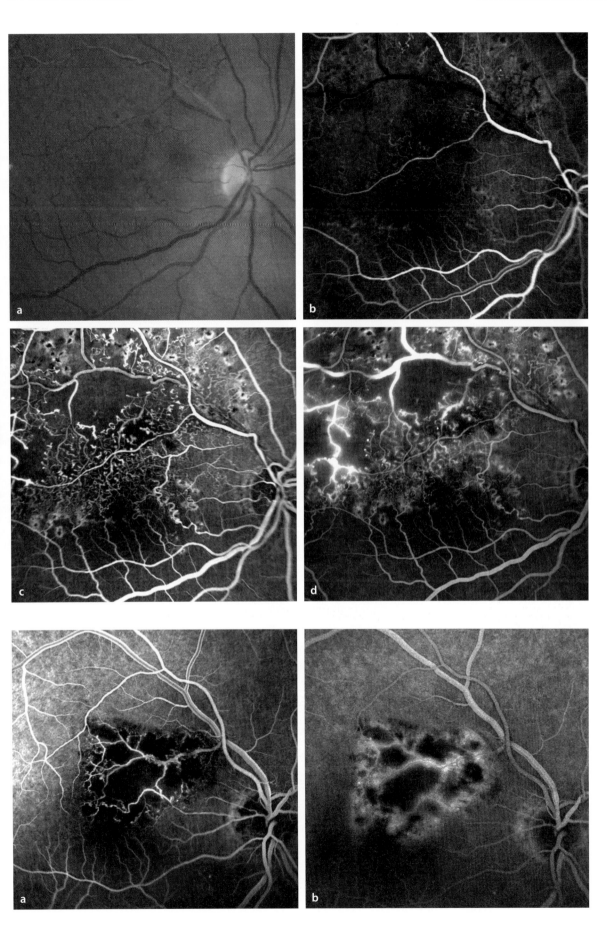

6.5   Retinal Macroaneurysms

Retinal macroaneurysms appear primarily in older patients that have a history of arterial hypertension. Women are more commonly affected than are men. There is a circumscribed dilation of a large retinal artery. In 10% of patients another macroaneurysm can be found in the contralateral eye.

Fundus

Retinal macroaneurysms are usually found along the superior or inferior retinal vascular arcades. As a result of damage to the vessel wall, one can often find retinal edema, hard exudates, and retinal hemorrhages. The aneurysm itself is often covered by these signs, making it difficult to identify. One can also find subretinal and intravitreal hemorrhages.

Fluorescein Angiography

In the arterial phase the macroaneurysm fills with dye. In some cases there is blockage of the background fluorescence by associated hemorrhages and exudates. An absence of hyperfluorescence in the area of the macroaneurysm suggests spontaneous thrombosis.

■ **Fig. 6.9a–c.** An 85 year old patient with a retinal macroaneurysm. **a** Fundoscopy shows a circumscribed vascular dilation in the inferotemporal artery with surrounding hemorrhages and a cotton-wool spot. **b,c** Fluorescein angiography makes identification of the macroaneurysm easy. The hemorrhages and cotton-wool spots block the background fluorescence. In the late phase some circumscribed leakage is seen around the macroaneurysm.

■ **Fig. 6.10a,b.** An 81 year old patient with spontaneous hemorrhage from a retina macroaneurysm. **a** Fundoscopy shows a retinal hemorrhage between the fovea the inferotemporal vascular arcade. A source of the bleeding is found in a circumscribed expansion of the arterial vessel. In addition there are parafoveal hard exudates. **b** Fluorescein angiography exposes the macroaneurysm. In the region of the retinal hemorrhage the background fluorescence is blocked.

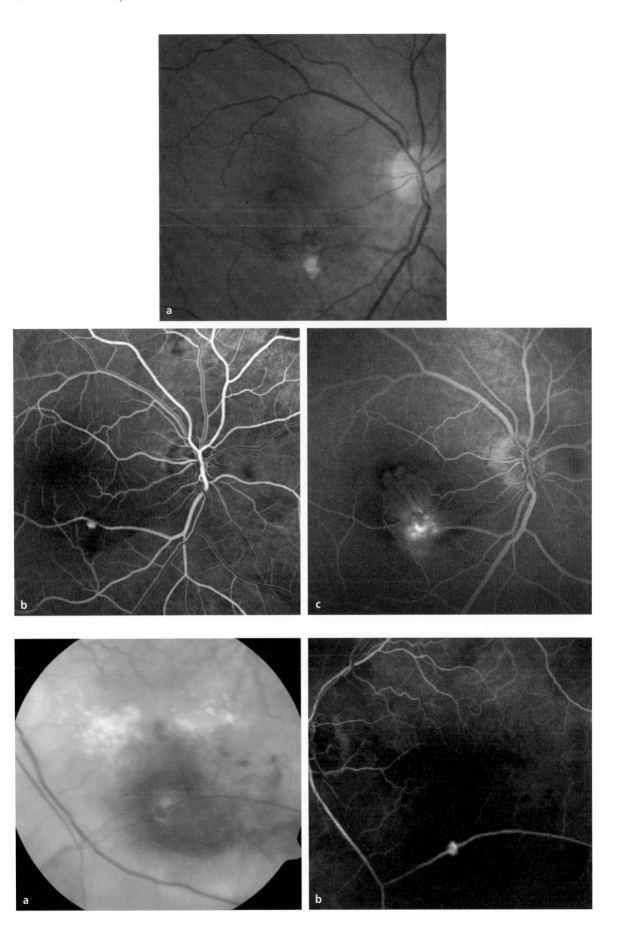

6.6 Coats' Disease

Coats' disease is a congenital retinal vascular anomaly that affects mostly boys. It is usually monocular. It is often first manifest between the ages of 4 and 10 years. The primary problem lies in an abnormal permeability of the capillary bed with marked exudation. In the affected retinal sectors one finds widening of the retinal capillaries and the larger retinal vessels, as well. There is also a thinning of the capillary bed. Massive exudation from both intraretinal and subretinal vessels can lead to a non-rhegmatogenous retinal detachment. The capillary occlusions can give rise to additional ischemic complications, including the development of neovascular glaucoma.

Fundus

There are widened retinal vascular segments, capillary ectasias, microaneurysms and often also large, circumscribed saccular expansions of vessels. The affected vessels are surrounded by flat, hard exudates and in some cases also flecks of surface hemorrhages. In advanced stages the massive subretinal exudation can lead to a complete retinal detachment.

Fluorescein Angiography

Fluorescein angiography reveals irregular expansion of retinal vascular segments. In the retinal periphery there are frequently areas with thinning of the capillary bed. At the margins of these hypofluorescent zones, one finds widened capillaries and also microaneurysms. During the later portions of the angiogram, leakage from the telangiectatic vascular segments. In the regions of hard exudates and hemorrhages the fluorescence phenomenon is blocked.

◘ **Fig. 6.11a–f.** A 14 year old patient with massive lipid exudation in the setting of Coats' disease. **a** Fundoscopy demonstrates flat, hard exudates, which in the fluorescein angiogram **b,c** lead to blockage of the background fluorescence. **d** In the retinal periphery are saccular changes in the retinal vessels are apparent.**e** Fluorescein angiography shows peripheral retinal areas, in which capillary perfusion is no longer present (i.e. areas of capillary non-perfusion). At the margins of these areas are telangiectatic capillaries. Also, saccular expansions of larger vessels can be seen. In the later course of the study **f** increasing leakage of dye from the affected vessel segments can be seen.

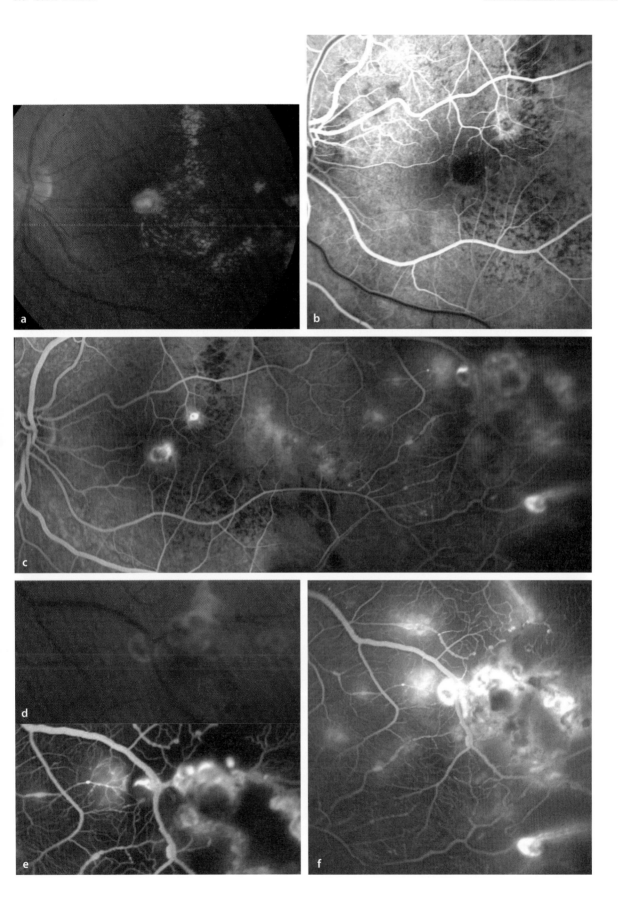

6.7 Retinal Capillary Hemangioma

Retinal capillary hemangiomas can appear sporadically, or in the context of the von Hippel Lindau syndrome. The latter is an autosomal dominantly inherited disease in which there is a genetic defect on chromosome 3 (locus 3p25). In the setting of this syndrome multiple retinal capillary hemangiomas can arise, there can be hemangiomas in the cerebellum and spinal cord, cyst formation in the pancreas, kidney and liver, and the appearance of a renal carcinoma. While the von Hippel Lindau syndrome can present with the appearance of multiple capillary hemangiomas in both eyes, in the sporadic form one more commonly finds a single, solitary capillary hemangioma. It appears as an orange-red, nodular tumor that grows endophytically (in the direction of the vitreous body) and is supplied with blood by retinal vessels. These tumors are initially small and can be difficult to distinguish from microaneurysms. Unmanaged, they grow slowly but continuously in size. The tumor is made up of proliferating capillaries and glial cells. With increasing size of the mass there is typically a marked increase in the sizes of the arterioles that feed and the venules that drain the growing tumor. Capillary hemangiomas become symptomatic when the accompanying exudation from the tumor, which increases as the tumor grows, deposits lipid exudates, causes macular edema and results in exudative retinal detachments. Glial cell proliferation can also lead to traction detachments of the retina. Retinal capillary hemangiomas are usually clinically manifest in the 2nd and 3rd decades of life and can also arise from within the tissues of the optic disc (▶ Chapter 8)

Fundus

It is a mostly red tumor of the retina, which is usually sharply margined. The retinal artery leading to the tumor and the retinal veins that drain it are dilated and have a tortuous course. The caliber of these vessels, in comparison to that of normal vessels, is several time larger. The tumor can be surrounded by hard exudates.

Fluorescein Angiography

During the angiogram, one can see the dye filling the retinal vessels and then the tumor itself. The tumor is completely hyperfluorescent. The veins draining the mass are likewise strongly hyperfluorescent. In the late phase the tumor can be seen to leak dye.

Fig. 6.12a–f. A 44 year old patient with the von Hippel Lindau syndrome. In both eyes retinal capillary hemangiomas have already been successfully treated with laser photocoagulation or cryopexy. Now the patient has presented with a newly arising retinal capillary hemangioma in the left eye inferior to the inferotemporal vascular arcade. In addition there is also a cerebellar hemangioma. **a** Fundoscopy shows a red colored, round tumor, which appears to rest on the retinal surface without disturbing the neighboring retina. The veins draining the tumor are dilated. At varying distances from the tumor are hard exudates of yellow lipid. **b–f** Fluorescein angiography: In the early phase **b** the arteriole supplying the tumor is filled with dye. This is followed by staining of the tumor, which appears completely hyperfluorescent. The two veins draining the tumor are dilated and sinuous. In the late phase there has clearly been leakage of fluorescein from the tumor **f**.

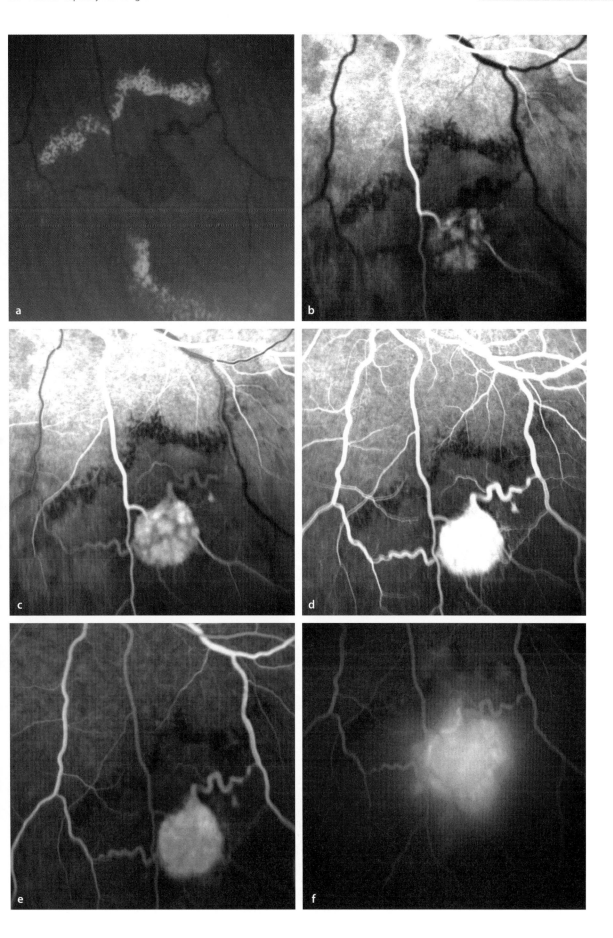

6.8   Cavernous Hemangioma of the Retina

Cavernous hemangioma of the retina is a rare hamartoma, i.e. an embryonal tumor containing disorganized retinal tissue components. The vascular tumor is usually located in the retinal periphery, however 10% of cavernous hemangiomas lie in the macular region and lead to loss of visual function. Cavernous hemangiomas of the optic disc have also been described. Peripheral cavernous hemangiomas are usually asymptomatic, although visual field testing of the affected area will find a scotoma. Inner, outer and intraretinal hemorrhages as well as vitreous hemorrhages have been described in association with cavernous hemangiomas, although they seldom lead to long term visual loss. As a rule, an increase in size of these embryonal tumors is not seen. Dermal and intracranial cavernous hemangiomas can be found in association with neuro-oculocutaneous syndromes (phakomatoses). Dermal hemangiomas are particularly common in the neck. Intracranial cavernous hemangiomas are usually found in the cerebrum and can cause seizures and intracranial hemorrhages. 40% of cerebral hemangiomas are calcified and can be seen in conventional X-rays. MRI scanning can detect uncalcified hemangiomas.

Fundus

There is an intraretinal collection of saccular aneurysms with telangiectatic and dilated vascular segments surrounded by glial tissue. The size of cavernous hemangiomas is usually less than two disc diameters

Fluorescein Angiography

Fluorescein angiography first shows a blockage of the background fluorescence in the area of the tumor. Since the vessel changes in a cavernous hemangioma arise from the capillary bed, they remain relatively isolated from the retinal circulation. Blood flow within the hemangioma is stagnant and staining of the saccular aneurysms by fluorescein progresses very slowly. Between the aneurysms are connecting, telangiectatic, dilated venules. Due to the very stagnant flow inside the aneurysms blood separates into its plasma and cellular components, meaning that the cellular elements sink, depending on their densities, while the superior portions of the aneurysms are filled with plasma. Correspondingly, the late phase shows pooling of fluorescein in the superior layers of the aneurysmal spaces. There is no leakage of dye, since the inner blood-retinal barrier usually remains intact.

■ **Fig. 6.13a–d.** A 47 year old patient with a cavernous hemangioma of the retina, which was discovered coincidentally. **a** Fundoscopy shows a glial tumor in the peripheral retina with widened vessel segments and numerous saccular aneurysms. **b,c** Simultaneous fluorescein angiography (*left image half*) and ICG angiography (*right image half*). The tumor blocks the background fluorescence. Also, the ICG angiogram shows that the choroidal vessels lying beneath the tumor are poorly defined. In the course of the angiogram there is a slow staining of the telangiectatic and swollen retinal vessel segments and of the aneurysms. **d** (*upper right*) In the late phase of the fluorescein angiogram one can see the full extent of the mass and the numerous aneurysms. Within individual aneurysms there is an erythrocyte-plasma separation with selective staining of the superior portions of the aneurysms.

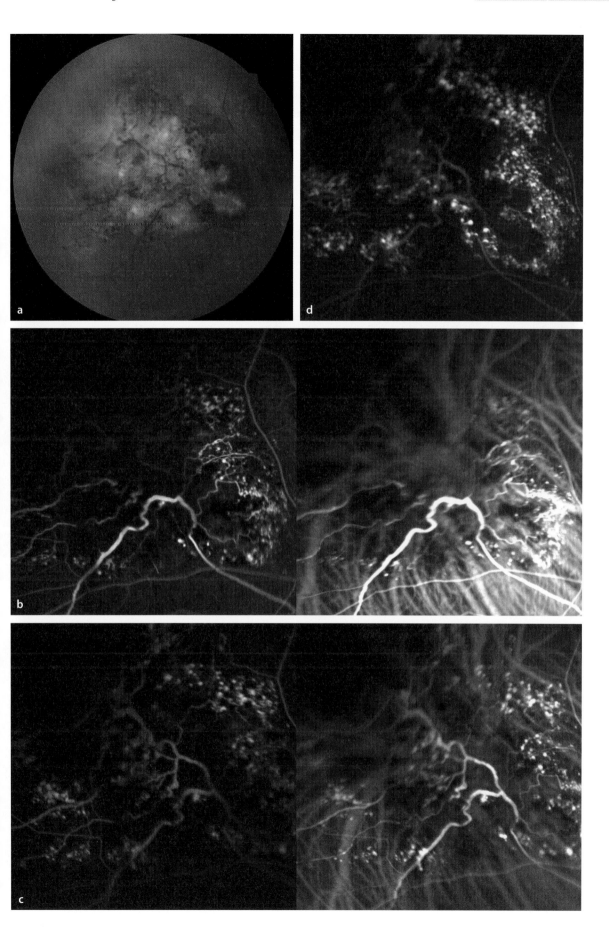

6.9   Vascular Tortuosity

Tortuosity or a pronounced, sinuous course of retinal vessels can be a component of many different congenital and acquired disorders. Congenital disorders include racemose hemangioma of the retina in which there are prominently dilated, large retinal vessels that extend from the optic disc with arteriovenous shunts. This anomaly can be associated with cerebral arteriovenous malformations. In this form it is referred to as the Wyburn-Mason syndrome. Congenital tortuosity can affect the entire retinal arterial tree. Unilateral cases of such findings suggest a congenital anomaly, as opposed to an underlying systemic disease. Bilateral tortuosity of the retinal vessels can be associated with cardiovascular diseases. Heart diseases that cause a chronic elevation of central venous pressure, chronic hypoxia, and an elevated hematocrit can cause the development of extremely tortuous retinal vessels. If cardiac function can be improved (e.g. a surgical procedure restores cardiac output) the tortuosity can regress.

Fig. 6.14a–f. A 22 year old patient with loss of vision in the right eye for 6 months (possibly much longer). The left eye appears unremarkable. The patient is otherwise healthy, and an MRI of the head has been reported to be normal. Visual acuity of the right eye is 20/40. A diagnosis of congenital retinal tortuosity has been made. **a,b** Fundoscopy shows pronounced tortuosity of the arterial retinal vessels. **c–f** Fluorescein angiographic imaging of the vascular anomaly. In the late phase **f** definite leakage of dye is seen from the perifoveal capillaries

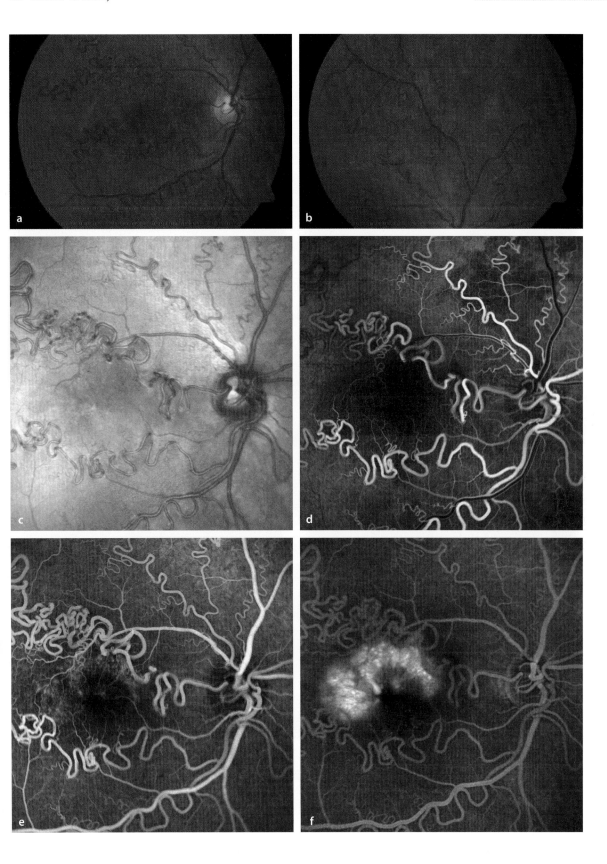

Inflammatory Retinal/Choroidal Disease

7.1   Toxoplasmic Retinochoroiditis

The basis for toxoplasmic retinochoroiditis is thought to be reactivation of an infection by toxoplasma gondii, acquired during the perinatal months of life. The consequence of a primary, perinatal infection is the formation of chorioretinal scars, which depending on their locations can lead to diminished visual function. Toxoplasma organisms can persist within tissues while in an inactive, encysted form. In the course of life, affected individuals can suffer a reactivation of this organism, presenting with the clinical signs of a posterior uveitis. Typically, the locus of reactivation can be found at the border of a primordial chorioretinal scar. Toxoplasmic retinochoroiditis can be complicated by the development of choroidal neovascularization.

Symptoms

Despite their locations, chorioretinal lesions of the fundus periphery often result in impaired vision, due to inflammatory loss of vitreous clarity

Fundus

Solitary or multiple, pale yellow, ill-defined foci, mostly without associated hemorrhages. Cellular infiltration of the vitreous, and frequently of the anterior chamber as well (◻ Fig. 7.1). After healing of the lesion, sharply margined chorioretinal scar.

Autofluorescence

While in the stage of active retinochoroiditis an elevated level of autofluorescence can be found. Autofluorescence in the subsequent chorioretinal scar is completely extinguished.

Fluorescein Angiography

Inflammatory damage to the blood-retinal barrier in the region of an active retinochoroidal lesion results in increasing leakage of dye. With regression of the inflammatory activity the leakage of dye seen during fluorescein angiography also diminishes. Post inflammatory chorioretinal scars are hypofluorescent. Angiography is particularly indicated when there is a suspicion of neovascularization.

◻ **Fig. 7.1a–f.** A 44 year old patient with visual acuity in the right eye of 20/200, caused by an active focus of toxoplasmic retinochoroiditis. **a** Fundoscopy finds a fluffy, white, paracentral focus of disease activity. Above the active lesion there are several sharply margined and irregularly pigmented chorioretinal scars. **d** Autofluorescence imaging shows an increased level of autofluorescence in the region of the active inflammation, while in the scarred foci the autofluorescence has been extinguished. **c** Fluorescein angiography shows at first a blockage of background fluorescence by the active inflammatory lesion. **d** During the angiogram there is clearly evidence of dye leakage, caused by damage to the blood retinal barrier. **e,f** The same patient one month later. While still on treatment, both the funduscopic and angiographic images show a regression of the inflammatory activity.

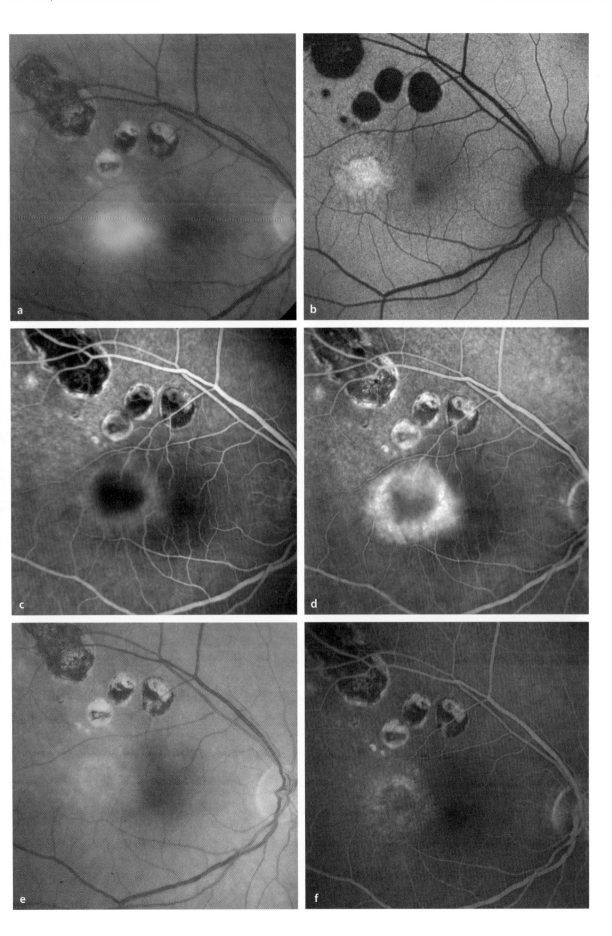

7.2   Multifocal Choroiditis

Multifocal chorioretinitis is a particular form of posterior uveitis with disseminated foci of inflammatory activity in the choroid and in some cases secondary involvement of the retina. Multifocal choroiditis belongs to the »white dot syndromes«, disorders that present with white inflammatory changes in the choriocapillaris. The etiologies can be manifold. The inflammatory foci heal with formation of chorioretinal scarring. Fluorescence angiography can be helpful in the diagnosis of active inflammatory lesions.

Fundus

Multiple chorioretinal scars and/or new foci of disease activity with white lesions in the choroid/retina

Autofluorescence

Autofluorescence is weak or missing in regions of chorioretinal scarring. The borders of scarred areas can present with elevated levels of autofluorescence.

Fluorescein Angiography

During the course of angiographic studies, well-healed, scarred foci appear as sharply margined hyperfluorescent areas without leakage of dye. In the vicinity of newly active inflammatory foci there is escape of fluorescein, caused by damage to the blood-retina barrier. These lesions have poorly defined margins due to the rapid escape of dye.

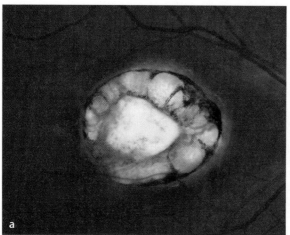

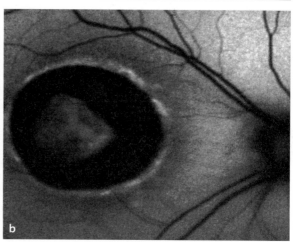

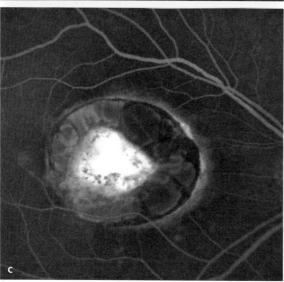

■ **Fig. 7.2a–c.** A 20 year old patient with a large chorioretinal scar in the posterior pole, probably the result of a prior bout of toxoplasmic retinochoroiditis. **a** Fundus image. At the border of the scar is a nearly circular line of hyperpigmentation, caused by RPE hyperplasia. Surrounding the center of the scar there is a band of tissue with no RPE and no choriocapillaris, so that one is looking directly at the large choroidal vessels. The center of the scar is completely white, since one is looking directly at the sclera. **b** Autofluorescence image. In the border zone of the scar there is a thin line of autofluorescence with an elevated level of intensity. At the center of the lesion the autofluorescence of the sclera is seen. **c** The late phase images of a fluorescein angiogram show hyperfluorescence in the area of sclera.

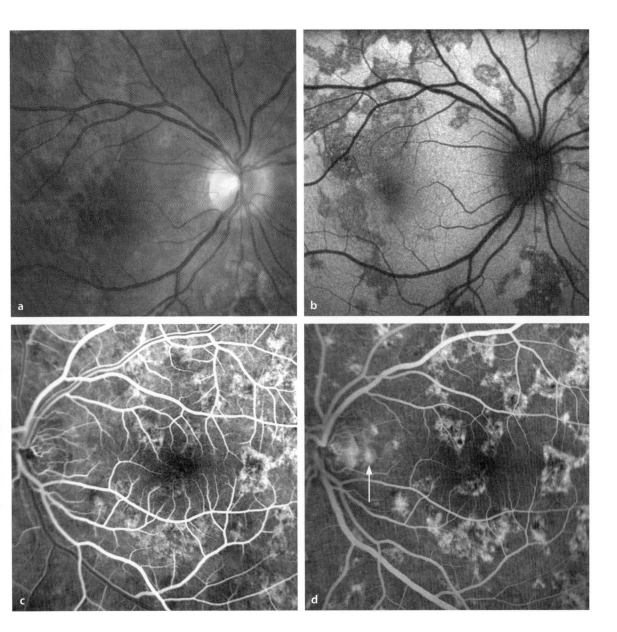

◻ Fig. 7.3a–d. A 14 year old girl with chronic, relapsing, multifocal choroiditis. **a,b** Fundus and autofluorescence images of the right eye show disseminated
patches of chorioretinal scarring. In the area of scarring the autofluorescence of the RPE is reduced or
completely gone, caused by the RPE atrophy. **c,d** The
early and late phase images from a fluorescein angiogram of the left eye show disseminated scars. Due
to the RPE atrophy, the scars are seen as hyperfluorescent (window defects). A small, active focus of inflammatory activity can be seen in the parapapillary
fundus. The inflammatory choroidal infiltrate causes
a block of the background fluorescence, while in the
late phase the same locations show circumscribed
areas of leakage (*arrow*).

7.3 Acute Posterior Multifocal Placoid Pigment Epitheliopathy (APMPPE)

APMPPE in young adults can develop following a viral infection, and belongs to the so-called »white dot syndromes« (see above). The cause is thought to be an immune vasculitis with disturbances of the circulaton in the choriocapillaris. This disease is usually bilateral.

Symptoms

Acute reduction in visual function, which in most cases improves spontaneously in a few weeks.

Fundus

In the posterior pole there are pale yellow flecks that are about one half of a disc diameter in size. The lesions appear simultaneously and evolve within a few weeks in parallel fashion to become more sharply defined and then atrophy into circumscribed, pigmented scars.

Autofluorescence

In the regions of inflammatory foci there is a reduction in autofluorescence. When healed, the locations of previously inflamed foci become strongly autofluorescent.

Fluorescein Angiography

In the early phase the lesions appear hypofluorescent, since the inflammatory foci block the choroidal background fluorescence. In the late phase the lesions develop a clear hyperfluorescence and stand out clearly against the background.

ICG Angiography

During ICG angiography the inflammatory foci, in both the early and the late phases, appear hypofluorescent. Usually, more lesion can be detected by ICG angiography than by fundoscopy.

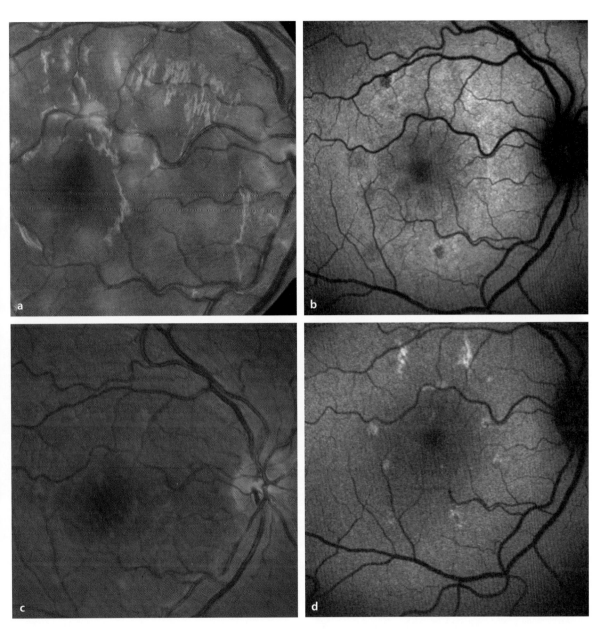

▫ **Fig. 7.4a–d.** A 26 year old patient with sudden onset of bilateral visual loss following a bout of gastroenteritis. **a** Right eye. There are multiple pale yellow lesions of APMPPE. Acuity 20/40. **b** Autofluorescence imaging: at the lesion sites there is a weakening of autofluorescence. **c** One month later the foci have completely healed with formation of small scars. Acuity has normalized. **d** The corresponding autofluorescence image shows an enhanced signal in the healed lesions, while the pattern of (previously) weakened autofluorescence can no longer be seen.

▶ **Fig. 7.5a–f.** A 32 year old patient with bilateral visual loss caused by APMPPE. **a** Fundoscopy finds pale yellow lesions at the level of the RPE that are mostly about one half of a disc diameter in size. In the left eye (not shown) there are identical changes. **b** In the locations of disease activity there is a reduction in autofluorescence. **c,d** Simultaneous fluorescein angiography (*left image*) and ICG angiography (*right image*): the lesions appear hypofluorescent due to blocking of the background fluorescence. In the late phase **d** a difference arises between the images of fluorescein versus ICG angiography – an FAG-ICG dissociation: while the lesions appear hyperfluorescent in the fluorescein angiogram, they remain hypofluorescent in the ICG angiogram. **e,f** Two months later the lesions have healed with formation of scars of varying size. During fluorescein angiography, the scarred lesions have a non-specific behavior, meaning that hyperpigmentation is associated with hypofluorescence, and areas of RPE atrophy are hyperfluorescent (window defects).

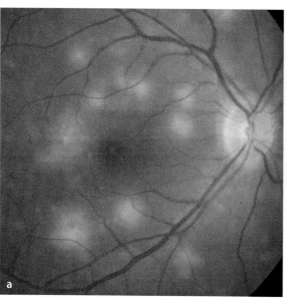

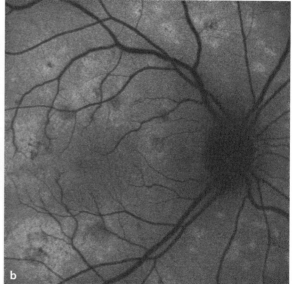

7.3 · Acute Posterior Multifocal Placoid Pigment Epitheliopathy (APMPPE)

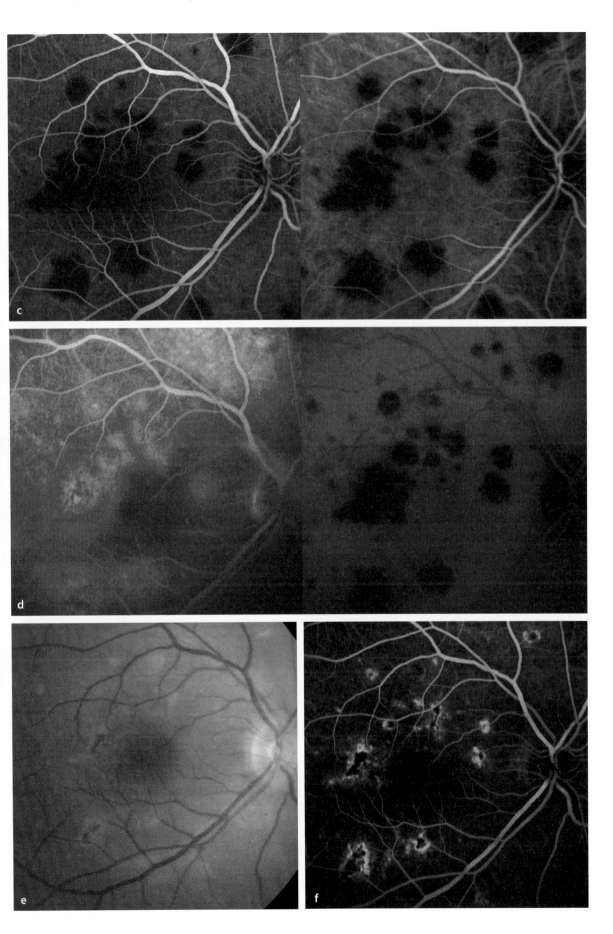

7.4   Punctate inner Choroidopathy (PIC)

Punctate inner choroidopathy (PIC) also belongs to the »white dot syndromes«. This disorder is uncommon and affects mostly young myopic women (peak age 15-40 years). Its etiology is not known. It can present as a monocular or binocular problem.

Symptoms

Reduced acuity and visual field defects (scotomas).

Fundus

There are pale yellow foci of inflammation in the posterior pole which have a size of about 100-300 μm and heal with scarring. Typically, there is no involvement of the anterior chamber or the vitreous body. The importance of this disease is that choroidal neovascularization can develop from the PIC lesions. The frequency of CNV involvement is estimated at about 40%, for which reason the prognosis of the disease is guarded.

Autofluorescence

In the area of scarred PIC lesions the autofluorescence signal is extinguished.

Fluorescein Angiography

In the early phase the PIC lesions can have a variable fluorescence pattern. In the scarred and healed lesions the choriocapillaris is damaged, so unlike a purely RPE atrophy there is no window defect with hyperfluorescence, rather there is hypofluorescence. In the late phase there is staining of the scarred PIC lesions, making them appear hyperfluorescent. The indication for fluorescein angiography is a suspicion of a possible CNV formation.

ICG Angiography

ICG angiography, as is typical in the »white dot syndromes«, clearly shows the areas of poor blood flow in the choriocapillaris. In the area of the lesions there is hypofluorescence

◘ **Fig. 7.6a–f.** A 31 year old myopic patient with unilateral PIC and prior photodynamic therapy of a secondary juxtafoveal CNV. **a** Fundoscopy finds numerous scarred PIC lesions in the posterior pole. Just superior to the fovea is a scarred, pigmented CNV. **b** Extinction of the autofluorescence signal at the various lesions. **c,d** Fluorescein angiography. The PIC lesions at first appear hypofluorescent, while in the later course of the study there is increasing leakage of dye. Also in the area of the treated CNV there is dye leakage without evidence of active CNV components. **e,f** The ICG angiogram shows the typical hypofluorescence of the PIC lesions caused by damage to the choriocapillaris. In the later course of the ICG study the hypofluorescent spots are particularly clear.

7.4 · Punctate inner Choroidopathy (PIC)

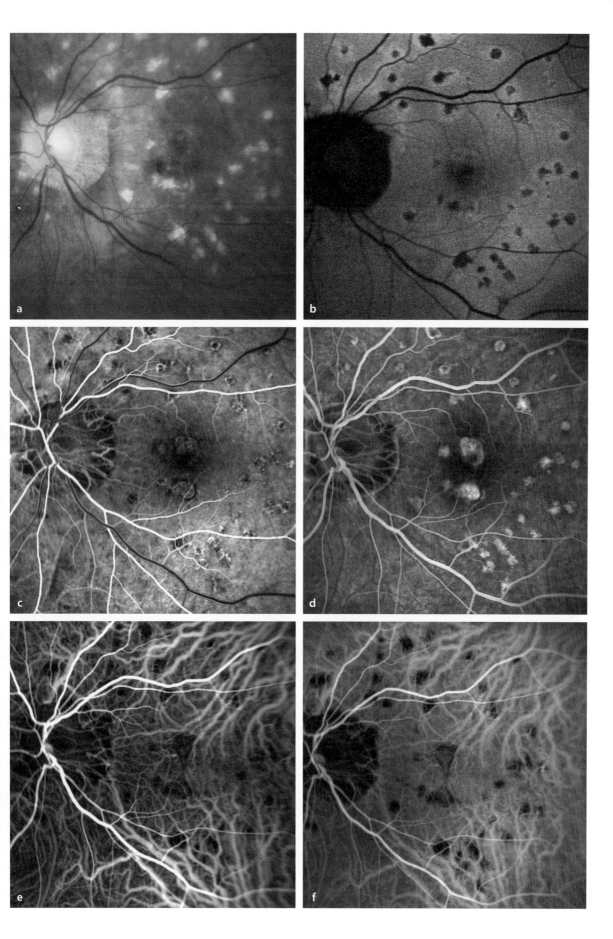

7.5 Presumed Ocular Histoplasmosis Syndrome (POHS)

Histoplasmosis is a fungal disease, acquired by inhalation of the spores of Histoplasma Capsulatum. This organism is known to be endemic in large areas of the United States. The acute phase includes flu-like symptoms, but no ocular involvement. A particular ocular finding (see below) has been ascribed to the fungus and is possibly an immune reaction. Presence of the fungal organism is very difficult to establish, and the clinical syndrome is also found in patients outside the USA, where the likelihood of exposure to Histoplasma C. is very low. One speaks therefore of a »presumed« ocular histoplasmosis syndrome (POHS). The diagnosis is difficult, but it is the ophthalmoscopic appearance that is decisive. The relevance of the disease is that POHS is a risk factor for the development of choroidal neovascularization.

Symptoms

POHS becomes symptomatic when there is development of choroidal neovascularization in or close to the macula.

Fundus

There are multiple zones of chorioretinal atrophy with a diameter of 0.2 to 0.6 disc diameters that have been called »histo spots«. These round flecks are white and can in varying degrees be hyperpigmented. There is no accompanying inflammatory reaction and no vitreous clouding. Additionally, a peripapillary zone of chorioretinal atrophy is frequently seen. In some cases a focus of choroidal neovascularization can be found that has originated in one of the lesions.

Autofluorescence

In the areas of atrophic lesions autofluorescence is frequently weakened or extinguished.

Fluorescein Angiography

During angiography the »histo spots« are easily identified as well-margined, hyperfluorescent foci. In the late phase the lesions can be particularly prominent due to their uptake of fluorescein (staining). Leakage can be found only when choroidal neovascularization has developed.

ICG Angiography

Due to choroidal atrophy in the areas of »histo spots«, they are hypofluorescent during ICG angiography.

Fig. 7.7a–f. A 46 year old patient in whom histoplasmosis was diagnosed 4 years ago. By history the last period of activity was 5 months ago. **a** In the right eye there are several sharp-margined, small round lesions (»histo spots«) that show a variable pigmentation. Also, there is a peripapillary zone of chorioretinal atrophy. **b** Blockage of autofluorescence at the histo spot locations. c,d Fluorescein angiography: Blockage of fluorescence correlating with areas of RPE hypertrophy within the spots, otherwise staining of the lesions becomes clear in the late phase. **c,d** Fluorescein angiography: Blockage of fluorescence correlating with areas of RPE hypertrophy within the spots. Staining of the lesions became clear in the late phase (**d**). **e,f** ICG angiography (**e**: middle phase; **f**: late phase). Easily seen are defects in the choroid (hypofluorescent zones) corresponding to the »histo spots«.

7.5 · Presumed Ocular Histoplasmosis Syndrome (POHS)

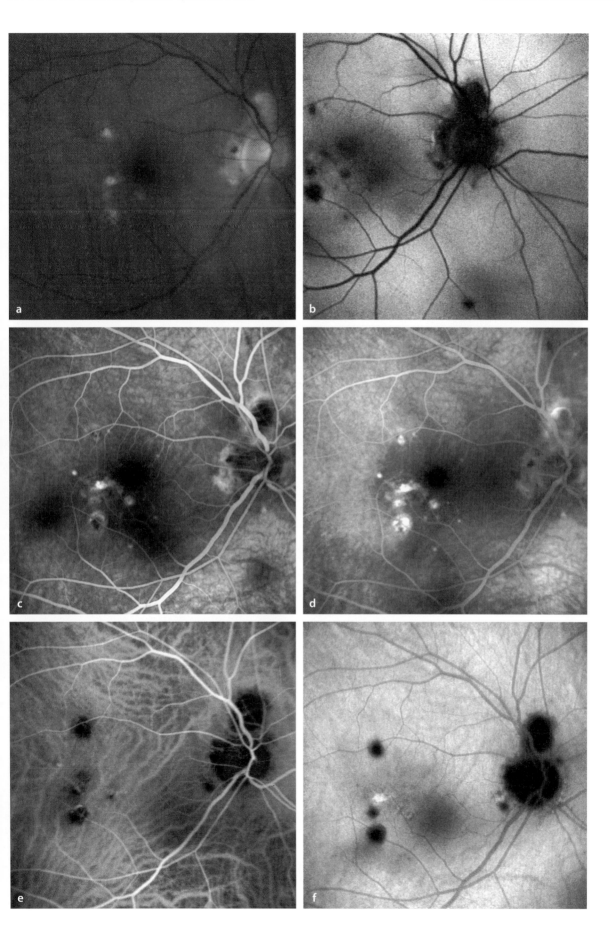

7.6   Birdshot Chorioretinopathy

Birdshot chorioretinopathy is a chronic, bilateral inflammatory disease that presents with characteristic funduscopic signs. It is an autoimmune disorder - up to 90% of patients are HLA-A29 positive. Some authors classify this disease among the »white dot syndromes«, while other authors do not classify it among the »white dot syndromes«, since it is not primarily an inflammatory disease of the choriocapillaris.

Symptoms

A reduction in acuity, caused by the associated vasculitis, cellular infiltration of the vitreous, and in some cases cystoid macular edema.

Fundus

Corresponding to the level of cellular infiltration, the vitreous clarity is reduced. There are striate, well margined, pale yellow areas of depigmentation. These changes appear follow the course of the deep choroidal vessels, and are most promi-nent in the nasal fundus. In addition, there can be vasculitis, vitreous cells and cystoid macular edema.

Autofluorescence

The autofluorescence levels change irregularly, and as a rule are they not diagnostically helpful.

Fluorescein Angiography

The characteristically striate lesions are only poorly visible on fluorescein angiograms. Corresponding to the extent of their associated vasculitis, there can frequently be both hyperfluorescence and leakage of dye in the vicinity of the large vascular arcades during the course of the study.

ICG Angiography

The ICG angiographic findings can include an irregular choroidal filling pattern. Compared to the extent of funduscopically visible lesions, however, the change in choroidal filling is low-grade. Clearly visible areas of hypofluorescence, as seen other »white dot syndromes«, are not found.

◻ **Fig. 7.8a–d.** A 65 year old HLA-A29 positive patient with birdshot chorioretinopathy. **a** Fundoscopy (left eye) shows depigmentation located nasal to the temporal large vessels with a well demarcated, pale yellow, striated appearance which is typical for this disease. The structures along the inferotemporal vascular arcade appear faded. **b** The autofluorescence image shows an irregular distribution of fluorescent intensity. **c,d** Simultaneous fluorescein angiography (*left half images*) and ICG angiography (*right half images*). The fluorescein angiogram shows hyperfluorescence, especially along the vascular arcades with increasing leakage of dye in the course of the study, while the ICG angiogram **d** is relatively unremarkable and shows no filling defects in the vicinity of the funduscopically visible changes.
(*For findings of the contralateral eye see* **e,f** *below*).

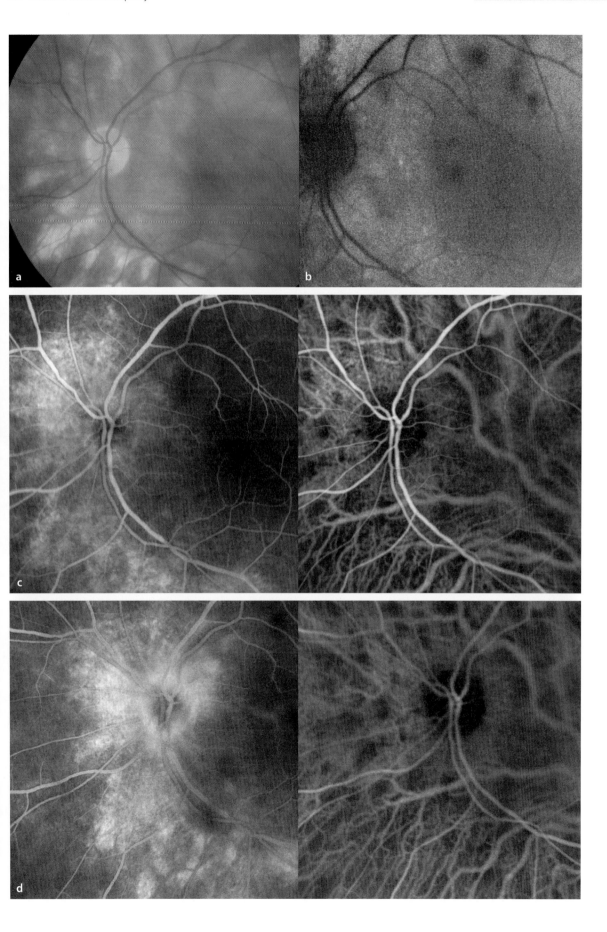

7

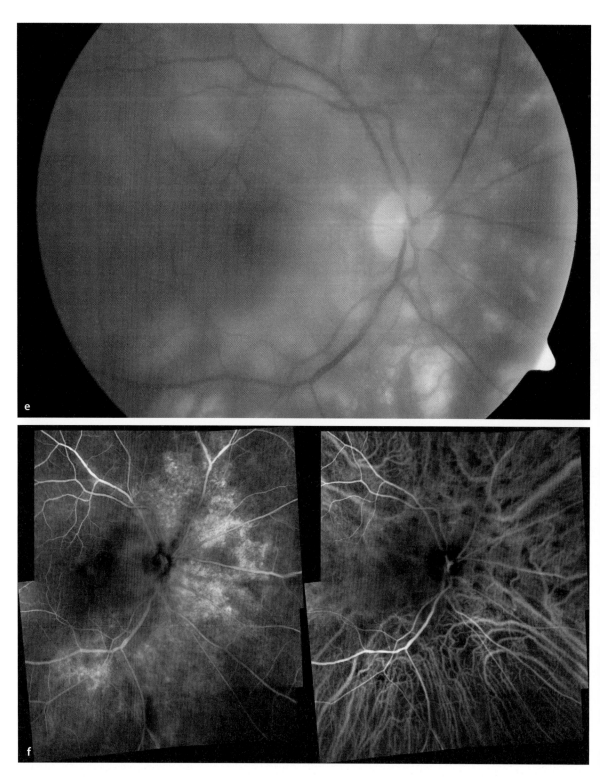

■ **Fig. 7.8.** *Continuation.* **e,f** A 65 year old patient with birdshot chorioretinopathy. Findings in the right eye are similar in appearance to those of the left eye. (**f** : simultaneous fluorescein/ICG angiography, composite images).

7.7   Perivasculitis

Perivasculitis retinae refers to an inflammation of the retinal vessels with vascular sheathing. The retinal veins are more frequently involved than are the arteries. Perivasculitis can be caused by any number of diseases. Among the group are sarcoidosis, collagenosis retinopathy, multiple sclerosis, and infections, such as tuberculosis, syphilis, and toxoplasmosis. In some patients the etiology remains unknown, often despite extensive diagnostic testing. It is assumed that these cases represent a form of autoimmune disease.

Fundus

Ophthalmoscopy shows off-white sheathing of the vessels, that as a rule appears only in portions of the arteries or veins, i.e. a segmental pattern.

Autofluorescence

In the area of sheathing there is an irregular blockage of autofluorescence, so that the affected vessel segments have indistinct margins.

Fluorescein Angiography

In the regions of the affected vascular segments there is an elevated permeability with leakage of fluorescein. This causes an increasing accumulation of dye that grows throughout the course of the angiogram.

ICG Angiography

Unlike the smaller molecules of fluorescein, the ICG molecules show no signs of leakage. The inflammatory changes in the affected vessel segments block the fluorescence somewhat, which is why the ICG fluorescence in these areas appears to remain confined to the intravascular blood columns.

7.7.1   Occlusive Retinal Vasculitis

Occlusive retinal vasculitis is a particular form of vascular wall inflammation which presents with vascular occlusions that lead to corresponding areas of retinal ischemia. Certain disorders, such as Behçet's disease (◘ Fig. 7.10) present with this type of vasculitis.

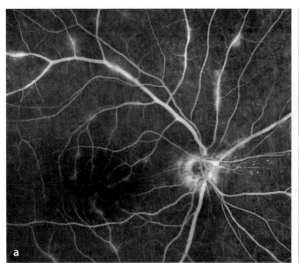 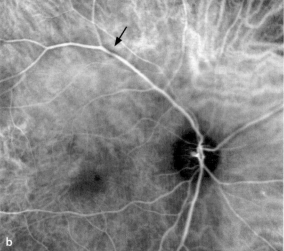

◘ **Fig. 7.9a,b.** A 45 year old patient with uveitis intermedia and multifocal periphlebitis. **a** Fluorescein angiography detects numerous retinal venous vascular segments with definite leakage of dye as a sign of segmental inflammatory damage to vascular wall permeability. **b** In the corresponding ICG angiogram there is no leakage. The zones of periphlebitis can cause blockage of the ICG fluorescence, and vascular wall edema can narrow the blood column to produce an hour-glass shaped restriction to blood flow (*arrow*).

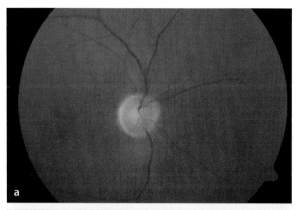

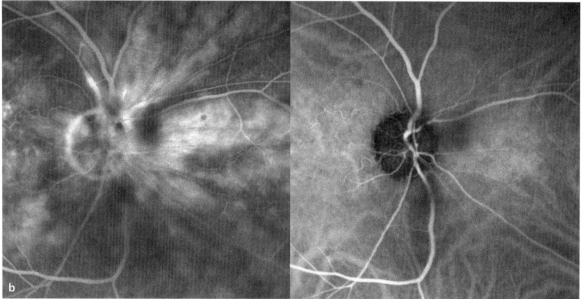

Fig. 7.10a,b. A 53 year old patient with the perivasculitis of Behçet's disease. **a** Long segments of sheathing of the peripapillary retinal arterial vessels. **b** Simultaneous fluorescein angiography (*left image*) and ICG angiography (*right image*): In the fluorescein angiogram there is in addition to a diffuse peripapillary leakage, a leakage of the superotemporal retinal artery superior to the optic disc, where this vessel is thickened, while the ICG study shows no leakage in this location.

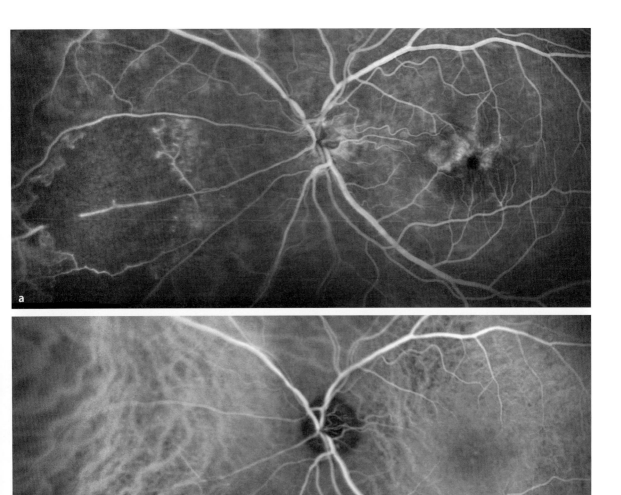

■ **Fig. 7.11a,b.** A 40 year old patient with occlusive retinal vasculitis of uncertain origin. The visual acuity of the left eye is 20/100. **a,b** Simultaneous fluorescein-ICG-angiography of the left eye. **a** Fluorescein angiography shows definite macular edema. Nasal to the optic disc is a circa 9 disc diameters wide area of retinal ischemia. There are abrupt retinal vascular terminations. **b** ICG angiography shows no damage to the choroidal circulation. The area of retinal ischemia is barely noticeable, due to the good visualization of the choroidal circulation. There is no leakage of ICG in the macula.

■ **Fig. 7.12a–f.** A 52 year old patient with bilateral occlusive vasculitis of uncertain cause. **a** Fundoscopy shows sheathing of the inferotemporal artery. **b–d** Fluorescein angiography shows a complete occlusion of the inferotemporal artery. The area supplied by this vessel is ischemic, the capillaries bordering on the area of ischemia are telangiectatic, and there is leakage of dye in the late phase **d. e,f** The right eye has paracentral retinal hemorrhages and cotton wool spots along the course of the superotemporal artery. Fluorescein angiography shows the broad area of ischemia.

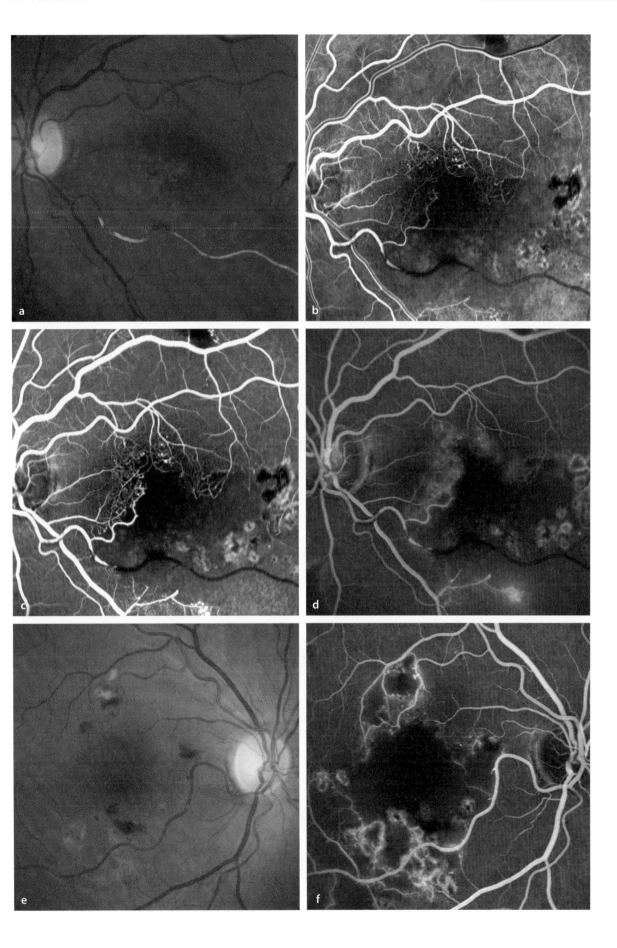

7.8   Inflammatory Macular Edema

Intraocular inflammation can lead to a generalized disturbance of the blood-retinal barrier in the regions fed by the retinal vessels and also in the outer retinal layers. This in turn can cause diffuse, cystoid macular edema.

Fluorescein Angiography

While the early phase of the study can be unremarkable, the middle phase shows a diffuse leakage of dye. In the late phase the extent of the macular edema is clearly recognizable. The angiographic findings often show the macular edema more impressively than the funduscopic findings might suggest.

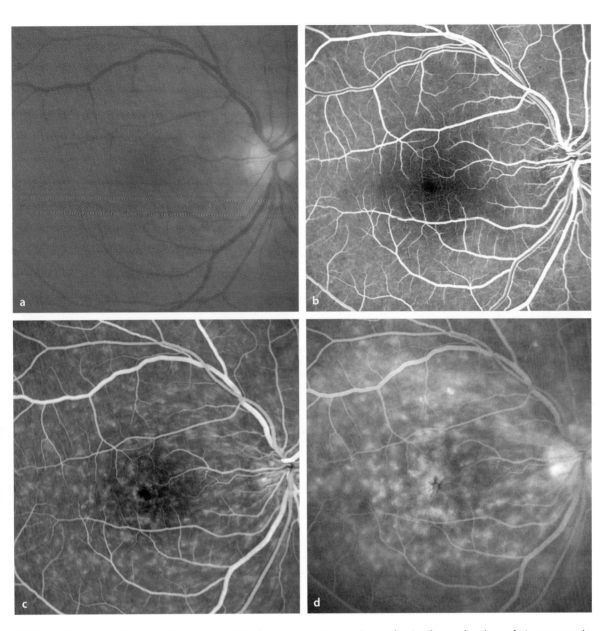

◘ Fig. 7.13a–d. A 30 year old patient with chronic, relapsing iridocyclitis for the past ten years, caused by a rheumatoid disease (Bechterew's, or Strümpell-Marie disease). The acuity in the right eye was 20/50. **a** Fundoscopy shows no unusual findings. Fluorescein angiography in the early phase **b** is unremarkable. In the subsequent course of the study **c** and in the late phase **d** there was a diffuse disturbance of the blood/retinal barrier with visualization of a pronounced level of macular edema.

7.9   Serpiginous Choroiditis

Serpiginous choroiditis is a disease of uncertain origin that causes damage to the choroid and the retinal pigment epithelium. As a rule, it affects both eyes.

Fundus

There are gray/white changes that typically extend from the optic disc and heal with scar formation. In the scarred areas of the choriocapillaris, the retinal pigment epithelium and the outer layers of the retina have been destroyed. The borders of the scarred areas of often bizarrely arcuate in shape (serpiginous). Newly active lesions extend from the borders of the scarred areas, causing them to grow ever larger. Also, choroidal neovascularization can arise at the margins of the scarred areas.

Autofluorescence

Autofluorescence is completely extinguished in the scarred areas.

Fluorescein Angiography

In the early phase new lesions block the background fluorescence. In the course of the angiogram leakage of dye appears in and around the active lesions. Frequently there are adjacent areas of scarring that appear hyperfluorescent, due to the atrophy of the retinal pigment epithelium. Since the choriocapillaris in the scarred area is also atrophic, the larger choroidal vessels are clearly visible.

▣ **Fig. 7.14a–f.** A 32 year old patient with an acute bout of serpiginous choroiditis in the left eye. **a** Fluorescein angiography in the early and mid phase show a hypofluorescent area the size of 5 disc diameters above the superior vascular arcade. This area corresponds to that of the active inflammatory lesions, which cause blockage of the background fluorescence. In the immediately adjacent areas there are hyperfluorescent scars which are the healed vestiges of prior inflammatory activity. **b** In the late phase diffuse leakage of dye appears in the region of active choroiditis. **c,d** The same patient 2 years later: large zone of atrophy of the RPE and the choriocapillaris at the location of the prior inflammation. The atrophic zone reaches all the way to the fovea; the acuity is 20/20. While on immunosuppressive therapy, there have been no additional bouts of inflammatory disease. **e,f** The right eye of the same patient shows a large area of scarring in the posterior pole, caused by prior activity of serpiginous choroiditis. Due to preservation of a small island that includes the fovea, acuity remains 20/20. The fluorescein angiographic appearance of an old, no longer active, serpiginous choroiditis is characteristic and is marked by the presence of a hyperfluorescent margin of scarring that retains its serpiginous shape.

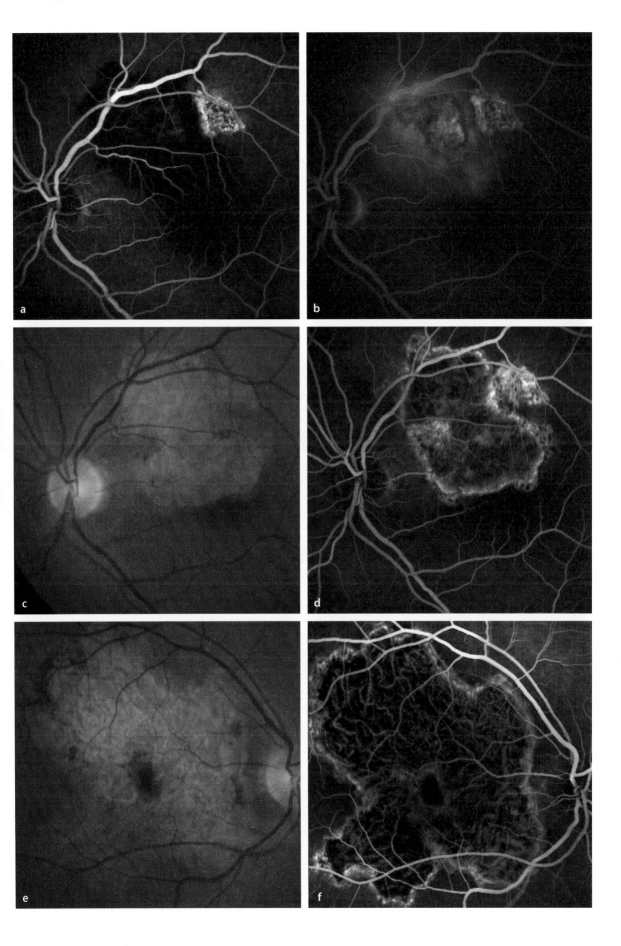

Diseases of the Optic Nerve Head

8.1 Congenital Anomalies of the Optic Disc

8.1.1 Oblique Insertion of the Optic Nerve

Oblique insertion of the optic nerve is typically seen as a tilting of the optic disc in an inferior or inferonasal direction. The disc appears unusually oval and the inferonasal quadrant of the disc is relatively pale. Frequently the temporal retinal vessels move at first in a nasal direction before turning about to sweep toward the temporal half of the fundus.

Fluorescein Angiography

The fluorescein angiographic appearance of an obliquely inserted optic nerve has no significant feature that differentiates it from an otherwise normal optic disc. With a pronounced degree of optic disc tilting the obliquely inserted optic nerve can be associated with an ectasia of the ocular wall, i.e. the ocular wall is thinned and drawn out in an inferonasal direction. This usually is found in company with a marked refractive error that makes parts of the fundus out of focus during the angiogram.

8.1.2 Myelinated Nerve Fibers

Myelinated nerve fibers are axons of the retinal ganglion cells which have acquired a myelin sheath, due to a developmental anomaly of myelin formation during the first months of life.

Fundus

A white, opaque coloring of the nerve fiber layer. Variation of the myelin formation along the individual nerve fibers causes the edges of the myelinated area to appear feathered or indistinct.

Fig. 8.1a–c. Oblique insertion of the optic nerve, left eye. **a** The optic disc markedly tilted inferonasally and with an oval shape. The temporal branches of the central retinal artery and vein initially move in a nasal direction when crossing the border of the disc, but then turn back to supply the temporal half of the fundus. There is an ocular wall ectasias inferonasal to the optic disc. **b,c** During confocal fluorescein angiography either the nasal **b** or the temporal **c** region of the fundus can be in focus, but not both.

Fig. 8.2a,b. a Myelinated nerve fibers at the superonasal margin of the optic disc. **b** The myelinated fibers block the fluorescence during fluorescein angiography.

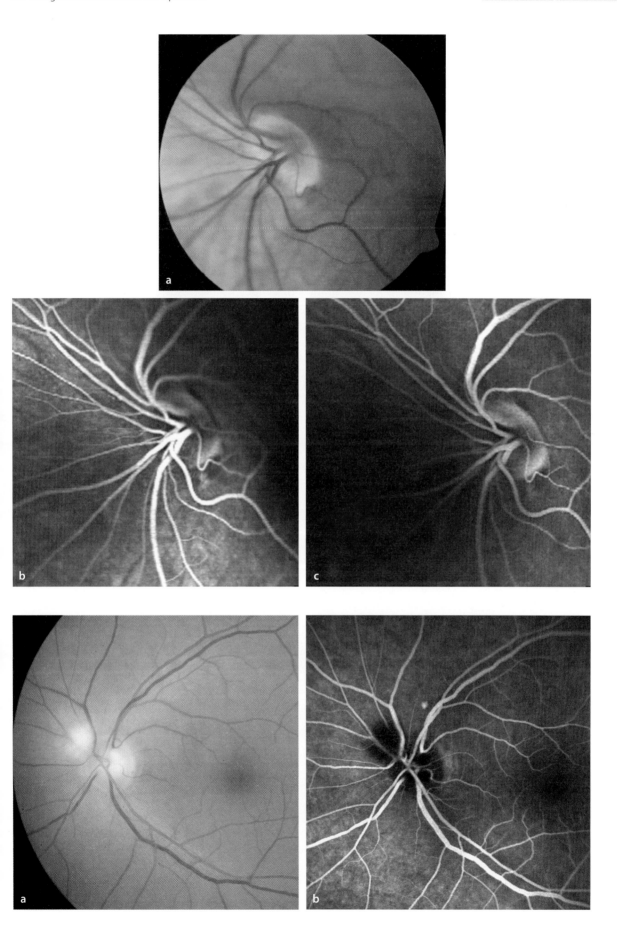

Autofluorescence / Fluorescein Angiography

The myelinated nerve fibers block both the auto-fluorescence and the background fluorescence phenomenon during angiography.

8.1.3   Drusen of the Optic Disc

Drusen of the optic disc are deposits of muco-polysaccharides, nucleic acids and calcium in the disc tissues (◨ Fig. 8.3). The scleral canal is normally narrow and the optic disc area is relatively small. Even though the papillary drusen usually remain asymptomatic throughout one's life span, some authors think they may be a cause of slowly progressive degeneration of the optic nerves. In children the drusen lie deep beneath the surface of the disc and are hard to find. During the second decade of life the drusen become visible as tiny, pearl-like, and elevated groups of spheres clustered together. Rarely, a parapapillary choroidal neovascular membrane is associated with drusen of the optic disc (◨ Fig. 8.4).

Symptoms

Optic disc drusen are usually asymptomatic. Occasionally, nerve fiber bundle defects appear in the visual field, corresponding to the course of the fibers damaged by the drusen. Such visual field defects usually do not reach the center of the field and are often not noticed.

Autofluorescence

The material deposited in the drusen is clearly autofluorescent. The autofluorescence of drusen is visible, only if they are prelaminar in location (anterior to the lamina cribrosa). Drusen in deeper tissues, as they some times develop in children, are not ordinarily visible by autofluorescence.

Fluorescein Angiography

Fluorescein angiography offers no additional advantage and is indicated only when there is suspicion of, for example, the presence of a choroidal neovascular membrane.

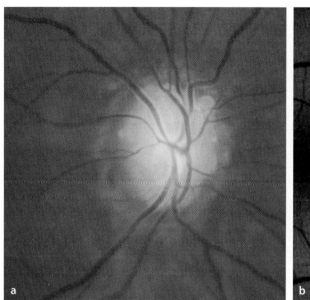 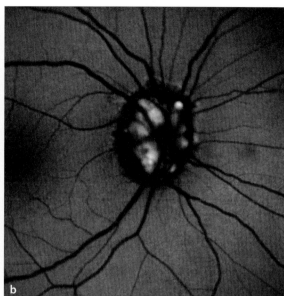

◨ **Fig. 8.3 a,b.** A 52 year old patient with optic disc drusen, which were discovered coincidentally. **a** Right eye. **b** The drusen show a distinctly elevated level of autofluorescence.

◘ **Fig. 8.4a–f.** Parapapillary choroidal neovavascularization in association with drusen of the optic disc. A 13 year old patient with a history of several months duration of symptomatic blurring of vision in the right eye. **a,f** Fundoscopy finds bilateral disc elevation with drusen. To exclude papilledema and a possibly elevated level of intracranial pressure, a cerebral MRI was done and the CSF pressure was measured. No signs of pathology were found. The right eye **a** has a lightly pigmented lesion located temporal to the optic disc with an appearance consistent with a long-standing, scarred focus of parapapillary choroidal neovascularization. Lipid exudation is seen particularly in the superior sector of the lesion. Temporal to the lesion is a disturbance with some atrophy of the RPE (*arrow*). Secondary RPE changes of this sort typically appear and are caused by chronic leakage of plasma into the subretinal space. **b** Autofluorescence imaging demonstrates several foci of elevated signal level in the region of the optic disc. **c–e** Fluorescein angiography reveals choroidal neovascularization with fluid leakage **e** temporal to the optic disc. The area of RPE atrophy is clearly marked as a zone of hyperfluorescence.

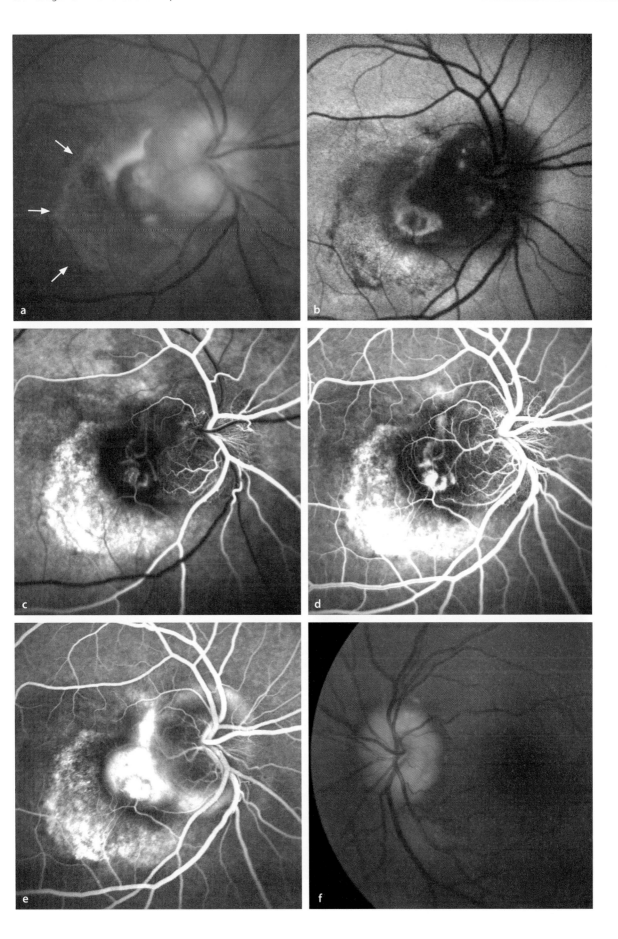

8.1.4 Coloboma of the Optic Disc

Colobomas are the consequence of failed closure of the fetal cleft of the optic cup. A coloboma of the optic disc is seen as an enlarged, deformed disc with a dysplastic excavation. The deepest part of the excavation usually lies in the lower half of the papilla. The exit of the retinal vessels is abnormal. Frequently there are anomalous peripapillary changes, seen as areas of hypo- or hyper- pigmention. Colobomas of the retina, choroid, lens, iris or lid can also be present (◘ Fig. 8.5).

Fluorescein Angiography

Due to the limited thickness of perfused tissues in the region of the coloboma, the region has a hypofluorescent appearance. The border of the papillary coloboma can be hyperfluorescent, however, caused by a retraction of the retinal pigment epithelium with transmission of the background choroidal fluorescence

8.1.5 Optic Pit

The optic pit is an anatomical defect in the parenchymal tissues of the papilla, and is usually located near the temporal margin of the optic disc. Occasionally there can be several pits. Fluid can leak from an optic pit into the subretinal space beneath the central retina with a resulting loss of vision (◘ Fig. 8.6).

Fluorescein Angiography

Angiography is usually not necessary in the management of an optic pit. However, when there is an associated detachment of the central retina, angiography will show a blockage of the background fluorescence by the subretinal fluid. A connection between the pit and the central area of detachment cannot be seen on an angiogram.

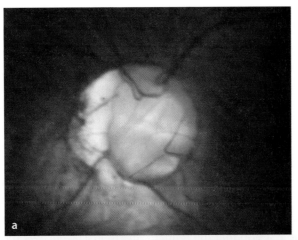

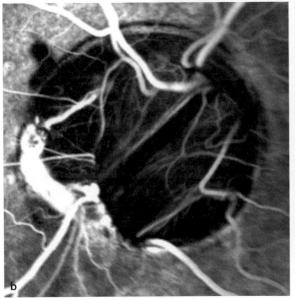

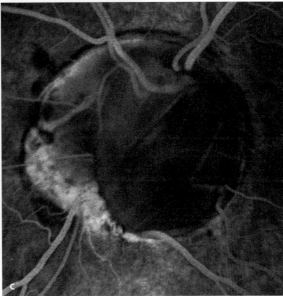

■ **Fig. 8.5a–c.** A 20 year old patient with a coloboma of the optic disc in the left eye. **a** Fundoscopy finds an enlarged optic disc surface area with a dysplastic excavation whose deepest point lies in the inferior half of the optic disc. **b,c** Fluorescein angiography of the colobomatous defect shows it to be hypofluorescent. Nasal to the optic disc is a scleral conus which due to the absence of the choriocapillaris also appears hypofluorescent. In the late phase **c** staining of the sclera is seen.

Fig. 8.6a–f. Optic pit with central retinal detachment. A 22 year old patient with a history of reduced vision in the right eye for the many months. **a** Fundoscopy shows a pit in the temporal quadrant of the optic disc at 9 o'clock. Temporal to this is a circumscribed pigmentation of the optic disc margin. Also, there is a central retinal detachment. Peripherally, one can see the transition between the still attached retina and the edematous, thicked but not yet detached retina (compare with the OCT). The actual retinal attachment is marked by the yellow ring of lipid. This ring lies at the transition from subretinal fluid to attached retina, and is a sign that the retinal detachment has been present for a long time. Centrally, one can see a cloverleaf-like, sharply margined zone in which the choroidal red appears to shine through more intensely. This effect is caused by a thinning of the central retina. **b** Infrared imaging shows the cloverleaf shaped area very clearly. **c,d** Fluorescein angiography (middle and late phases): Blocking of the background fluorescence by the retinal detachment, and increased transmission of the fluorescence in the area of central retinal thinning. **e** The OCT section through the optic disc shows the pit-shaped excavation in the temporal sector of the papillary tissue. **f** In the area of the macula, the central retinal detachment is seen with thinning of the retinal layers near the center of the detachment. Toward the pit (right side of the image) intraretinal edema can be clearly seen.

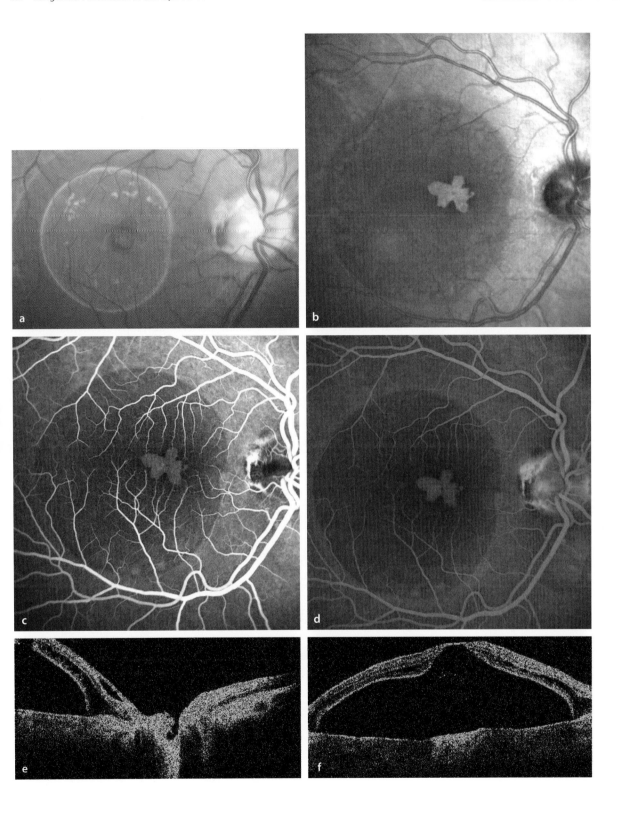

8.1.6 Capillary Hemangioma of the Juxtapapillary Retina

Capillary hemangiomas of the retina (▶ Chapter 6) can also present in the juxtapapillary retina and then extend to the optic disc. This form of retinal capillary hemangioma can present either in the setting of the von Hippel Lindau syndrome or as a solitary lesion. It is believed that it is a congenital malformation, despite the fact that hemangiomas often clinically manifest first among adults. They are therefor hamartomas, i.e. embryonal tumors arising from persistent rests of tissue. Unlike peripheral hemangiomas, such as those in the von Hippel Lindau, they have no large, dilated vessels to supply and drain their blood. By exudation and growth in size these tumors become symptomatic, with the clinical manifestations frequently first appearing between the second and third decades of life. While peripheral capillary hemangiomas (▶ Chapter 6) are usually endophytic (grow inward in the direction of the vitreous), juxtapapillary hemangiomas can have **endophytic**, **exophytic** or **sessile** growth patterns.

8.1.6.1 Endophytic Growth

A juxtapapillary capillary hemangioma presents as a redish, sharply margined tumor on the surface of the juxtapapillary retina (◨ Fig. 8.7). The vascular architecture of a hemangioma is recognizable. Vessels leading to or from the tumor are not visible.

Fluorescein Angiography / ICG Angiography

With filling of the retinal circulation the vessels of the hemangioma are immediately evident. In the further course of the study the tumor acquires a homogeneous hyperfluorescence, since the fluorescein molecules exit the intravascular space to enter the tissues of the tumor. ICG angiography, on the contrary, does not show this pattern, since the ICG molecules remain intravascular. In the late phase signs of leakage of fluorescein become evident, extending beyond the borders of the tumor.

8.1.6.2 Sessile Growth

This growth pattern develops in hemangiomas located in the middle and external layers of the retina (◨ Fig. 8.8). Clinically, the tumor can appear gray and flat. The large retinal vessels pass over the tumor. There can be an associated serous detachment of the retina with lipid exudation. When there is macular involvement, the differential diagnosis should include optic disc edema with a parapapillary choroidal neovascular membrane.

Fluorescein Angiography

The sessile hemangioma also appears together with the retinal circulation. Vessels within the hemangioma are initially defined before the entire tumor becomes hyperfluorescent. The associated serous detachment of the retina is barely noticeable. While the hemangioma has a fine capillary net, the vessels within a choroidal neovascular lesion are arranged primarily in a radial fashion (Differential diagnosis of parapapillary CNV, ▶ Chapter 8.5).

◨ **Fig. 8.7a–f** *(Figure parts e and f are located on the following page.)* A 58 year old patient with no symptoms. Coincidental discovery of a juxtapapillary retinal capillary hemangioma of the right eye. **a** Schematic diagram of the hemangioma's location. **b** Fundoscopy shows the endophytic growth pattern of the hemangioma, which sits on the papillary and retinal surfaces. **c–f** Simultaneous fluorescein/ICG angiography. Demonstration of the tumor's own vascular structure together with the retinal circulation. The hemangioma appears homogeneously hyperfluorescent with subtle leakage in the late phase. ICG angiography on the contrary shows the dye filling the tumor with a less pronounced and inhomogeneous pattern. The late phase **f** shows that the fluorescein molecules have left the intravascular compartment to enter the tumor tissues, while the ICG angiogram shows no such movement of the dye.

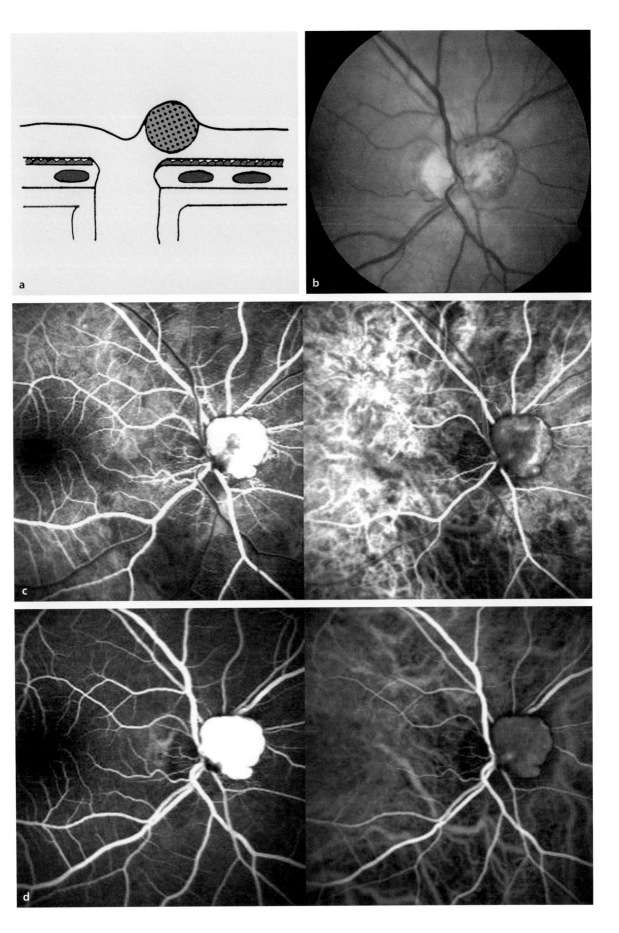

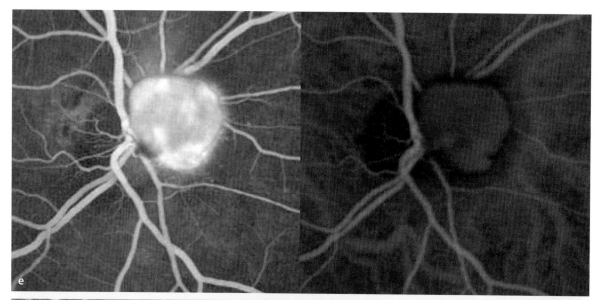

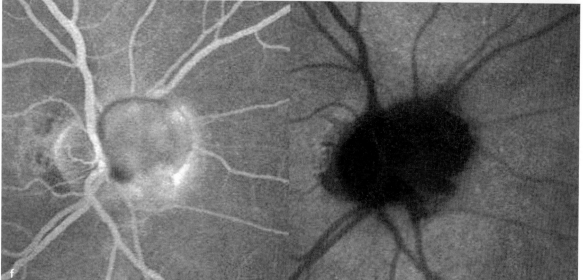

◘ **Abb. 8.7.** *Continued.*

◘ **Fig. 8.8a–f.** A 26 year old patient with a juxtapapillary retinal capillary hemangioma of the sessile type. Visual acuity of the right eye reduced to 20/200. The patient is otherwise in good health. **a** Schematic diagram of the hemangioma's location. Fundoscopy shows the tumor as a gray thickening of the retina nasal to the optic disc from 1 to 5 o'clock (*arrow heads*). From this location there is a flat, serous detachment of the retina (*arrows*) that is surrounded by a ring of yellow exudate. This lipid accumulation is especially prominent in the macula. **c–f** Fluorescein angiography demonstrates the vascular network of a juxtapapillary capillary hemangioma together with the retinal circulation. During the study the tumor becomes homogeneously hyperfluorescent through escape of the fluorescein molecules into the tissues of the tumor. In contradistinction to the endophytic growth pattern, the flat, intraretinal location of the hemangioma is apparent from the undeviating passage of the retinal vessels over the surface of the tumor's retinal location. The retinal capillaries located above the tumor are somewhat dilated. In the region of the subretinal lipid accumulation there is a blockage of the background fluorescence. In the late phase **f** the associated serous detachment of the retina is scarcely visible.

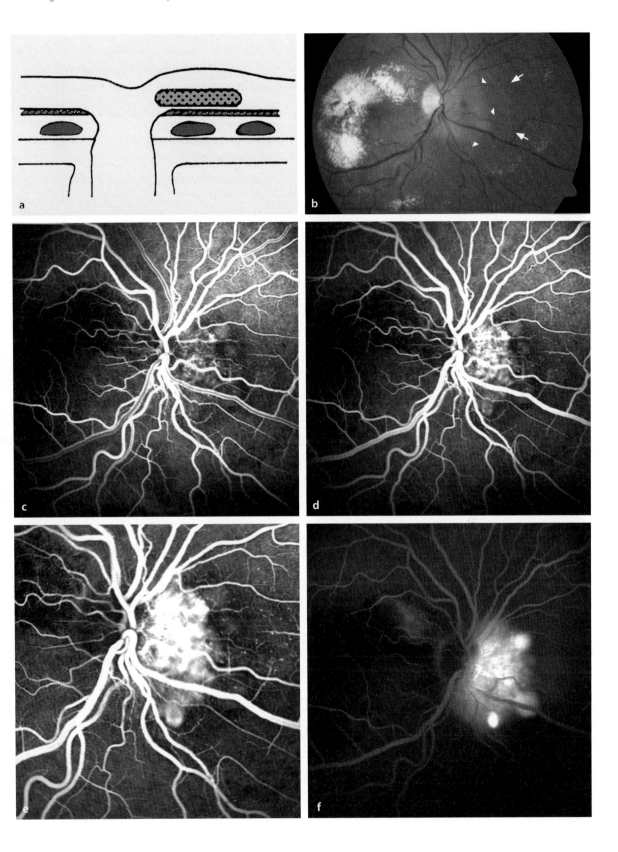

8.1.6.3 Exophytic Growth

The exophytic growth pattern of a juxtapapillary capillary hemangioma is well marked by the fact that the growing tumor takes its exit from the outer layers of the retina, and then grows beneath the retina. Clinically this tumor appears as a prominent, red-orange, intra- and subretinal tumor over which the retinal vessels pass. One occasionally sees superficial, dilated retinal vessels that lead outward, passing into the tumor. This growth pattern is also associated with the formation of serous retinal detachments with accumulation of lipid exudates.

Fluorescein Angiographie / ICG-Angiography

The fluorescein angiographic appearance of these tumors corresponds to the growth patterns described above.

■ **Fig. 8.9a–f.** A 57 year old patient with a juxtapapillary capillary hemangioma of the exophytic type. Acuity in the right eye reduced to 20/50; the patient otherwise in good health. **a** Schematic diagram of the hemangioma's location. **b** Fundoscopy shows a red, prominent, rather sharply margined tumor just nasal to the optic disc. The tumor is primarily subretinal and is surrounded by a flat, serous retinal detachment with subtle lipid exudation. **c** Autofluoresence image: In the area of the hemangioma there is a blockage of the normal autofluorescence. **d** ICG angiography clearly demonstrates the hemangioma. **e** Fluorescein angiography demonstrates the hemangioma together with the retinal circulation. In the late phase **f** leakage of dye can be seen surrounding the hemangioma.

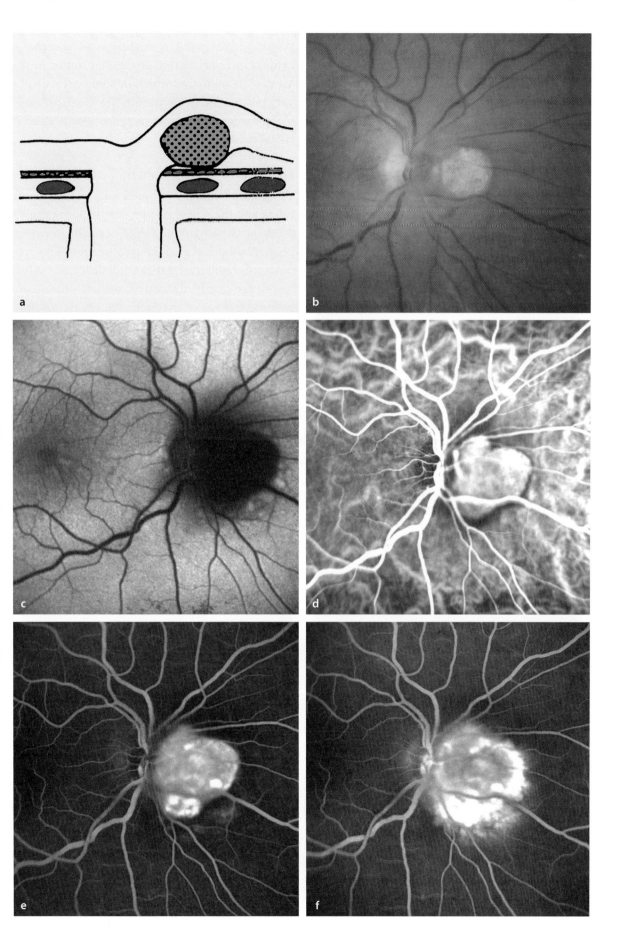

8.1.7 Pigmented Optic Disc Anomalies

the congenital, pigmented anomalies of the optic disc include the juxtapapillary combined hamartoma of the retina and pigment epithelium and the melanocytoma, a very uncommon, pigmented hamartoma. These two benign entities must be distinguished from the uveal melanoma with optic disc involvement.

Fundus

The juxtapapillary combined hamartoma of the retina and the retinal pigment epithelium is an irregular pigmentation in the region of the optic disc and the surrounding retina with glial proliferation and vascular ectasias. The changes are sharply margined and relatively flat. Glial cell proliferation and hyperpigmentation are found on the retinal vessels, which can be partially obscured and distorted by the process. The melanocytoma is a very darkly pigmented tumor in the area of the optic disc which in some cases can be very prominent. In contrast to the uveal, parapapillary, malignant melanoma, there is no peripapillary retinal detachment.

Fluorescein Angiography

The juxtapapillary, combined hamartoma of the retina and the retinal pigment epithelium causes a blockage of background fluorescence by its hyperpigmentation and glial cell proliferation. The pronounced capillary ectasias and distorted retinal vessels are clearly revealed. In the late phase there is some leakage of dye from the ectatic vascular segments. The melanocytoma also causes a blockage of the normal papillary fluorescence. Contrary to the uveal malignant melanoma, the malanocytoma has no intrinsic vascular structure.

Fig. 8.10a–d. A 44 year old patient with coincidental discovery of a juxtapapillary combined hamartoma of the retina and retinal pigment epithelium in the left eye. Acuity 20/20. **a** Fundoscopy finds delicate pigmentation and glial cell proliferation in the region of the optic disc and the peripapillary fundus. The peripapillary vessels are distorted, which becomes clearly apparent **b–d** during fluorescein angiography. In the late phase there is a subtle leakage of dye coming from the distorted vascular segments.

Fig. 8.11. A 23 year old patient with a melanocytoma of the optic disc (right eye). There is a flat, rather dark pigmentation with no associated serous retinal detachment. These findings have been stable for 5 years. The patient has no vision problems; the acuity is 20/20.

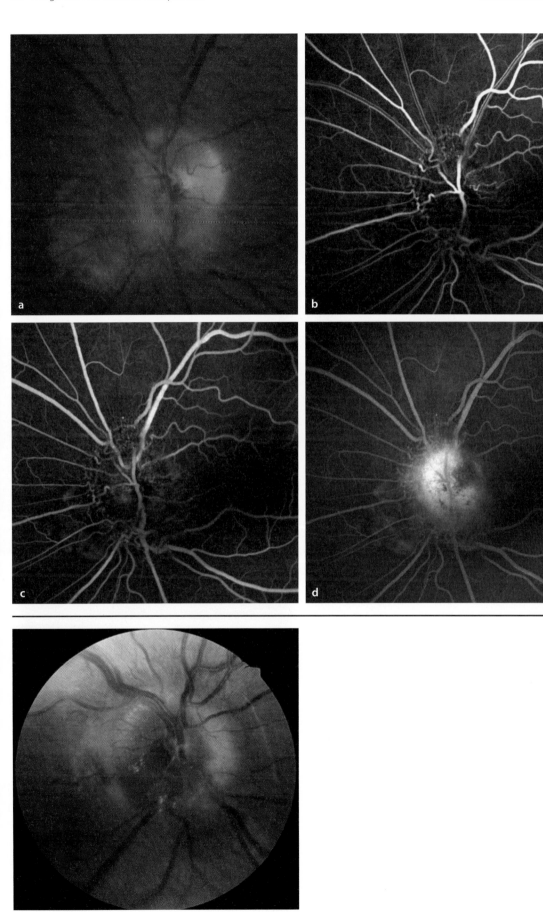

8.2   Anterior Ischemic Optic Neuropathy

Anterior ischemic optic neuropathy (AION) is the result of a failure of perfusion of the prelaminar optic disc. Underlying problems can be primarily arteriosclerotic or inflammatory processes (temporal arteritis). The hypoxic damage to axoplasmic flow causes swelling of the ganglion cell axons: papilledema. Depending on the severity of the process, splinter hemorrhages can appear in the nerve fiber layer.

Autofluorescence / Fluorescein Angiography
The swollen axons cause a blockage of both the autofluorescence and the peripapillary background fluorescence. Perfusion of the optic disc can be delayed. In the area of papilledema there are capillary ectasias. In the late phase there is leakage of dye into the swollen tissue of the optic disc.

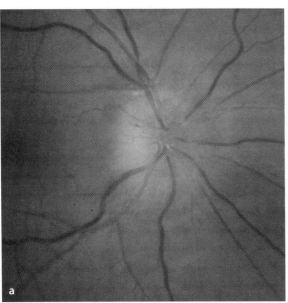
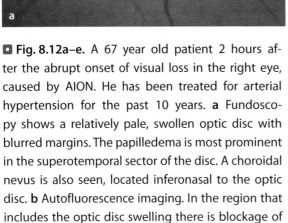
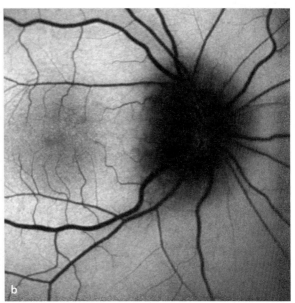

◻ **Fig. 8.12a–e.** A 67 year old patient 2 hours after the abrupt onset of visual loss in the right eye, caused by AION. He has been treated for arterial hypertension for the past 10 years. **a** Fundoscopy shows a relatively pale, swollen optic disc with blurred margins. The papilledema is most prominent in the superotemporal sector of the disc. A choroidal nevus is also seen, located inferonasal to the optic disc. **b** Autofluorescence imaging. In the region that includes the optic disc swelling there is blockage of the autofluorescent phenomenon. **c–e** Simultaneous fluorescein angiography (*left half images*) and ICG angiography (*right half images*): The disc swelling blocks the peripapillary background fluorescence. In the early phase there is a delayed perfusion of the optic disc, particularly in the superotemporal sector. There are dilated capillaries on the surface of the optic disc. In the late phase **e** of the fluorescein angiogram there is leakage of dye which is bounded by the area of optic disc swelling.

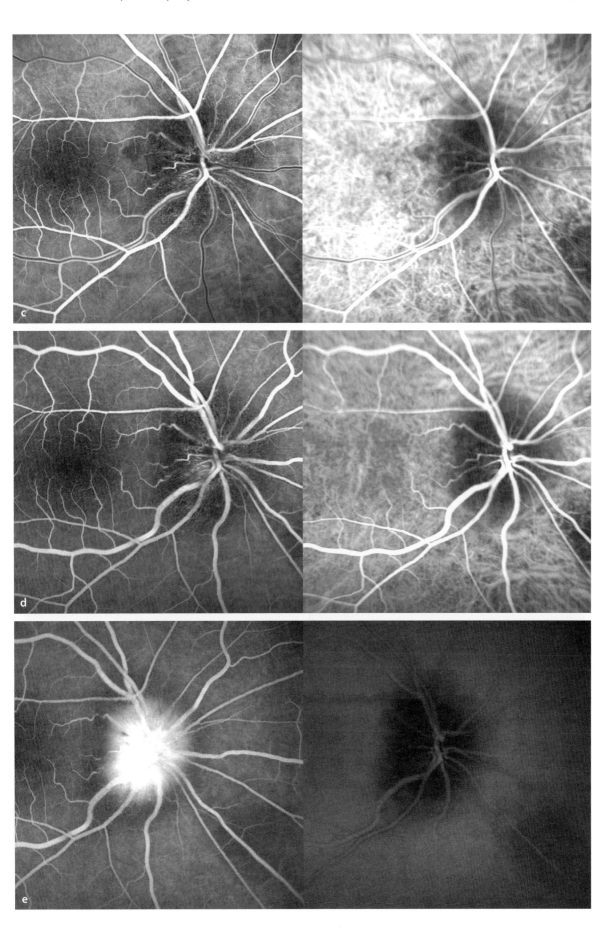

8.3   Papillitis

Papillitis is a circumscribed inflammation of the optic disc that has a highly varied group of possible underlying causes. Clinically there is a blurring of the margin and a prominence of the optic disc. The swelling of the disc tissue can interfere with blood flow in the retinal vessels, leading to central retinal vein occlusion.

Autofluorescence / Fluorescein Angiography

In the region of disc edema there is a reduction in the normal autofluorescence signal and during fluorescein angiography there is a blockage of the normal background fluorescence. During the course of the angiogram dilated capillaries appear on the surface of the disc. The late phase shows leakage of dye bounded by the swollen disc.

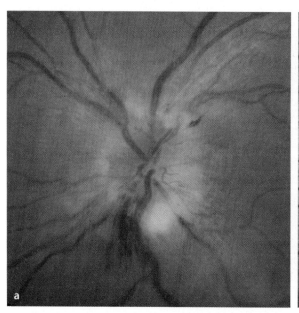
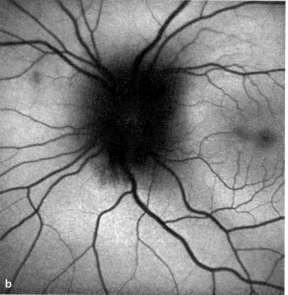

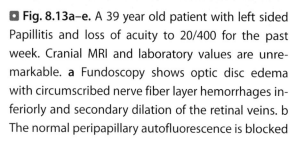

☐ **Fig. 8.13a–e.** A 39 year old patient with left sided Papillitis and loss of acuity to 20/400 for the past week. Cranial MRI and laboratory values are unremarkable. **a** Fundoscopy shows optic disc edema with circumscribed nerve fiber layer hemorrhages inferiorly and secondary dilation of the retinal veins. **b** The normal peripapillary autofluorescence is blocked in the area of disc edema. **c–e** Simultaneous fluorescein angiography (*left half images*) and ICG angiography (*right half images*): In the course of the angiogram there are increasing numbers of telangiectatic and altered capillaries in the region of disc swelling. In the late phase there is demonstration of fluorescein leakage bounded by the edematous disc.

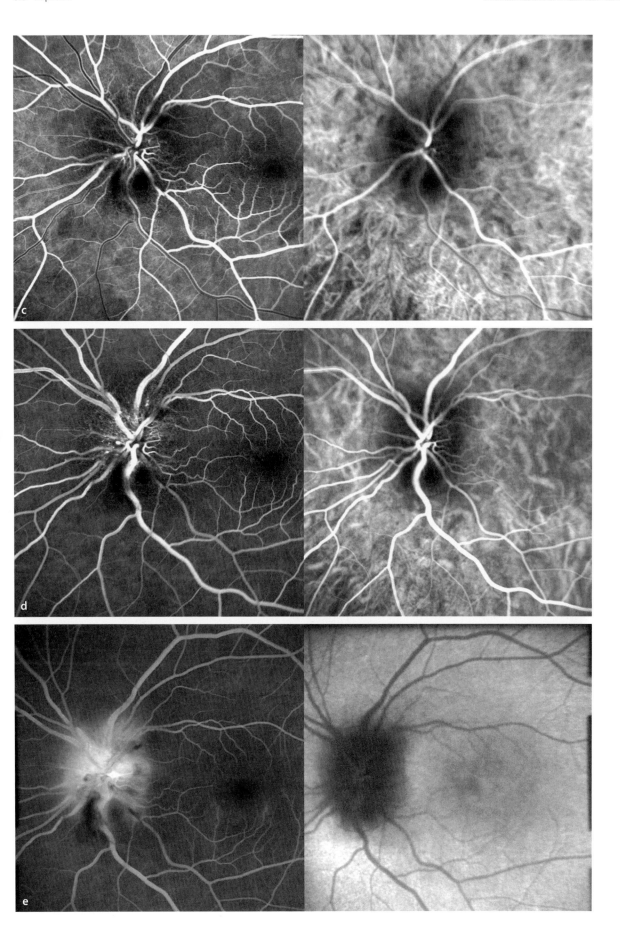

8.4   Papilledema

Papilledema arises when there is elevation of the intracranial pressure. The associated elevation of pressure in the optic nerve sheaths leads to interference with axoplasmic flow, the consequence of which is a swelling of the axons. The swelling of the optic disc tissues causes the neuroretina to be displaced, causing an enlargement of the physiological blind spot.

Autofluorescence / Fluorescein Angiography

Papilledema leads to a reduction of the normal peripapillary autofluorescence signal and in the fluorescein angiogram it leads to a blockage of the background fluorescence. Angiography shows the dilated capillaries in the swollen disc tissue, and in the late phase there is leakage of dye bounded by the edematous disc.

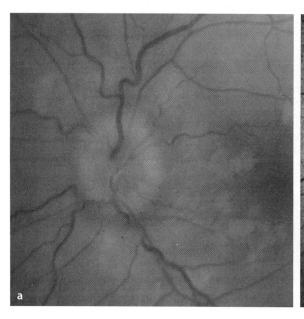
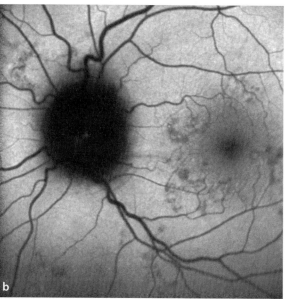

◻ Fig. 8.14a–e. A 52 year old patient with pseudotumor cerebri and bilateral papilledema. Acuity has been reduced to in both eyes to 20/30. **a** Left eye: distinct papilledema with blurring of the disc margins and dilation of the central veins. Associated findings include isolated perimacular zones of RPE atrophy. **b** Autofluorescence imaging: The optic disc margins are blurred, since the papilledema in part blocks the normal parapapillary autofluorescence.

c–e Simultaneous fluorescein angiography (*left half images*) and ICG angiography (*right half images*): During the angiogram there is demonstration of dilated capillaries on the surface of the swollen optic disc. **d** An associated finding are hyperfluorescent zones correlating with the areas of RPE atrophy. In the late phase **e** fluorescein leakage appears in the region of the swollen disc tissue.

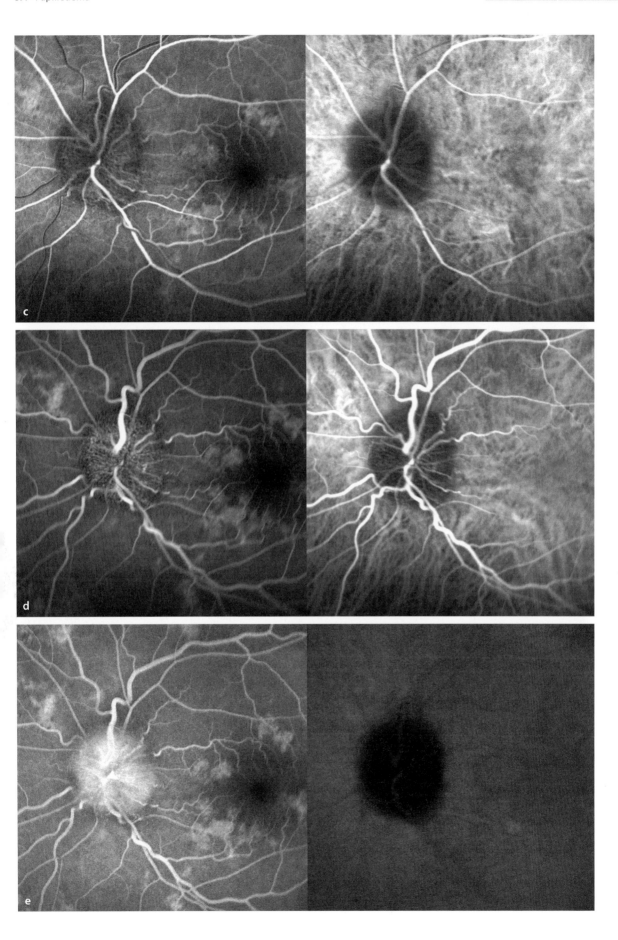

8.5 Parapapillary Choroidal Neovascularization

Choroidal neovascularization (CNV) can arise directly at the margin of the optic disc, and the temporal side of the disc is the usual point of departure in formation of a CNV membrane. There are many known predisposing factors. These include age-related macular degeneration (▶ Chapter 5), angioid streaks (▶ Chapter 5), optic disc anomalies (▶ Chapter 8.1), and prior inflammatory disease activity (POHS, chorioretinitis, ▶ Chapter 7).

Symptoms

The disease is particularly noticed by the patient when fluid exudation originating in the CNV reaches the region of the papillomacular bundle, extending to the foveal retina.

Fundus

At the papillary border there appears a prominent gray-white subretinal lesion that is in varying degrees accompanied by subretinal hemorrhages and surrounded by lipid exudation. The neighboring margin of the optic disc is often blurred.

Fluorescein Angiography

As in the CNV lesions that occur in other locations (▶ Chapter 5) there is a parapapillary CNV that is hyperfluorescent during the course of the angiogram. In the late phase there is a clearly visible leakage of dye from the CNV lesion.

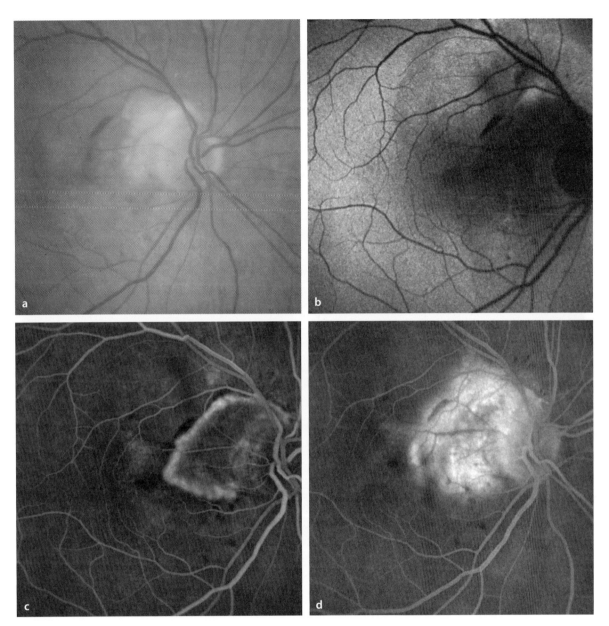

Fig. 8.15a–d. A 70 year old patient with para-papillary CNV in the right eye. **a** Fundoscopy shows temporal blurring of the optic disc margin, caused by an exudative subretinal process temporal to the optic disc. Isolated subretinal hemorrhages are visible. The process is bounded by a pigmented line that extends to the fovea. **b** Autofluorescence imaging shows a blockage of the normal autofluo-rescence in the region of the CNV. **c** Fluorescein angiography shows a clearly defined choroidal neo-vascular membrane temporal to the optic disc. The CNV shows the elements of a classic CNV (▶ Chapter 5.1.4.1) with a hyperfluorescent margin and a small neighboring zone of hypofluorescence. In the late phase **d** there is clearly visible leakage of dye from the CNV membrane.

Intraocular Tumors

The most common intraocular tumors are choroidal melanoma and choroidal metastases. Tumors arising from retinal blood vessels are described in ▶ Chapter 6. Elevation of the optic disc is covered in ▶ Chapter 8.

9.1 Choroidal Melanoma

Choroidal melanoma is the most common primary intraocular malignancy among adults. The clinical appearance of these tumors can be quite variable and is dependent on the degree of pigmentation in the tumor, the presence of »orange pigment« on the tumor's surface, and secondary changes in the RPE overlying the tumor. Also important are unusual growth patterns like the so-called collar button melanoma, in which a portion of the tumor grows through Bruch's membrane into the subretinal space.

Fluorescein Angiography

Corresponding to the variability of clinical findings, the fluorescence phenomenon in choroidal melanomas is also variable. If there is no significant blocking of fluorescence by heavy pigmentation, and depending on the pattern of vascularization in the tumor, filling of the choroidal vessels is accompanied by a hyperfluorescent appearance within the tumor. This is mostly irregular and appears clearly during the course of the study due in part to blockage of some of the background fluorescence and a variable degree of dye leakage in the area of the mass.

ICG Angiography

ICG angiography has the potential to image smaller vessels within a tumor's own vascular network. Although ICG angiography would appear to be an ideal candidate for such studies, in practice it has not be very effective and cannot reliably answer questions regarding a tumor's intrinsic vascular structure.

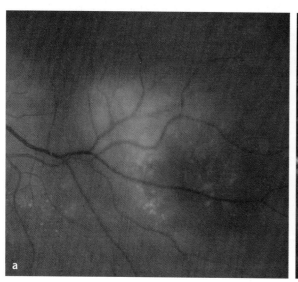 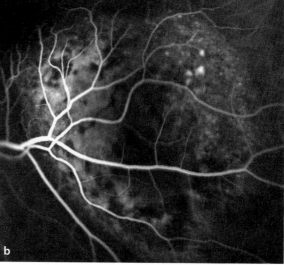

■ **Fig. 9.1a,b.** A 79 year old patient with a choroidal melanoma in the left eye. **a** Fundoscopy shows a partly amelanotic and partly pigmented tumor in the region of the inferotemporal vascular arcade.

b Fluorescein angiography shows a mottled hyperfluorescence within the tumor that increases during the course of the study.

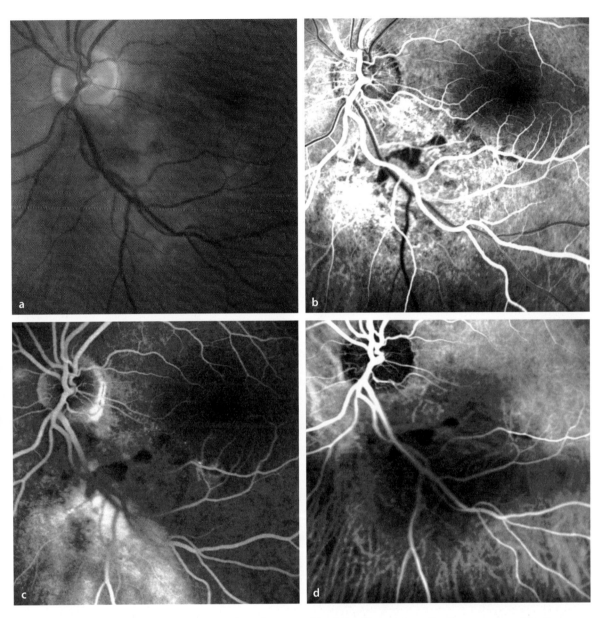

■ **Fig. 9.2a–d.** A 56 year old patient with a choroidal melanoma in the left eye. **a** Fundoscopy shows a prominent melanocytic choroidal tumor inferotemporal to the optic disc and extending into the macula. The tumor is partly pigmented; in the middle of the tumor are circumscribed zones of RPE hypertrophy. **b** With filling of the choroid, fluorescein angiography shows an irregular hyperfluorescence. The hypofluorescent flecks correspond to the zone of RPE hypertrophy. **c** In the late phase there is an adjacent (hyperfluorescent) zone of subretinal exudation inferior to the tumor. **d** In the ICG angiogram one can see within the tumor a disruption of the regular choroidal vascular architecture. Vessels that are clearly intrinsic to the tumor cannot be identified.

9.2   Choroidal Metastases

The most common primary tumor with choroidal metastases is carcinoma of the breast, which has usually been recognized long before its appearance in the eye. The second most common primary tumor is bronchogenic carcinoma. Choroidal metastases manifest as individual or multiple flat to elevated masses, usually posterior to the equator of the globe.

Fluorescein Angiography

Angiographic images correspond with the manifold variations of clinical signs seen in the fundus.

The early phase shows primarily blocking of the background fluorescence, causing the metastases to appear hypofluorescent. In the late phase irregular areas of hyperfluorescence appear. In very prominent metastases, an intrinsic vascular architecture can be identified.

ICG Angiography

ICG angiography of metastatic tumors usually shows areas of hypofluorescence, since the metastases interfere with or block the filling of choroidal vessels. These areas of hypofluorescence are mostly apparent in the late phase, but occasionally there are also flecks of hyperfluorescence.

◻ **Fig. 9.3a–f.** A 39 year old patient with a metastasizing adenocarcinoma. There are multiple metastases; the location of the primary tumor could not be identified. **a** Large choroidal metastases in the right eye. **b** Corresponding infrared image. **c,d** Simultaneous fluorescein angiography (*left half images*) and ICG angiography (*right half images*). The retinal vessels passing over the prominent metastases are out of the plane of focus and appear blurred. An intrinsic vascular network could not be demonstrated. In the late phase there are fluorescein angiographic foci of hyperfluorescence without leakage, while ICG angiography shows hypofluorescence produced by displacement or blockage of choroidal vessels remains unchanged. **e,f** In the left eye are also metastases with an identical angiographic pattern. (**f**: ICG angiography).

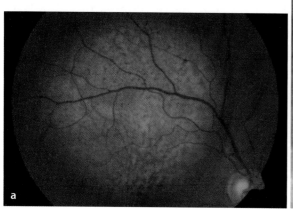

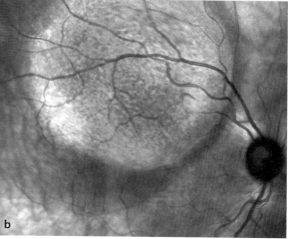

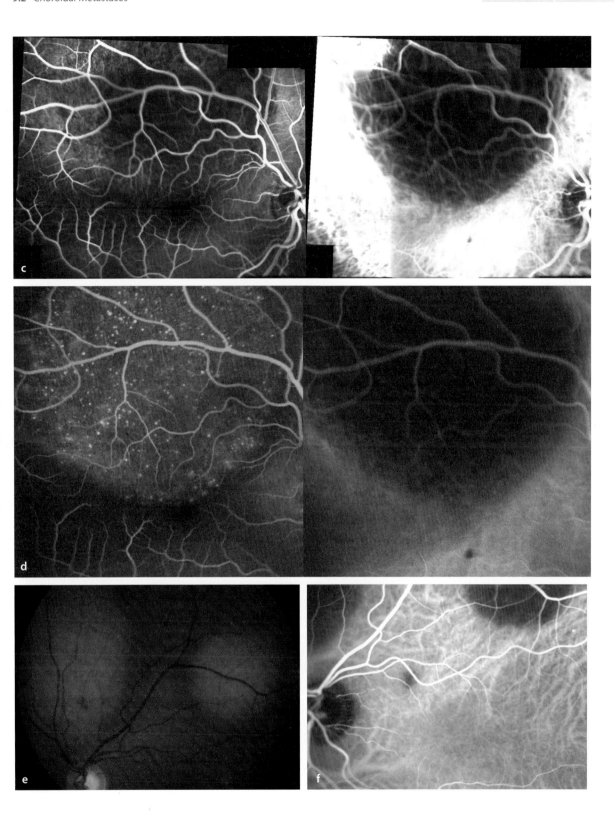

Fig. 9.4a–d. A 60 year old patient with choroidal metastases from a bronchogenic carcinoma. **a** Fundoscopy of the right eye shows a centrally located, prominent, solid choroidal tumor, which has echographic features consistent with a metastatic carcinoma. **b** Autofluorescence imaging shows an irregular pattern in the tumor region, and at the nasal border of the tumor is also a wrinkling of the choroid that parallels the border of the tumor. **c,d** Simultaneous fluorescein angiography (*left half images*) and ICG angiography (*right half images*). In the region of the tumor's prominence the retinal vessels leave the plane of focus. The normal background fluorescence is blocked. In the course of fluorescein angiography numerous point-like foci of hyperfluorescence appear **d**. In the ICG angiography there is a blocking of the fluorescence in the choroidal circulation. There is no indication of an intrinsic vascular structure.

9

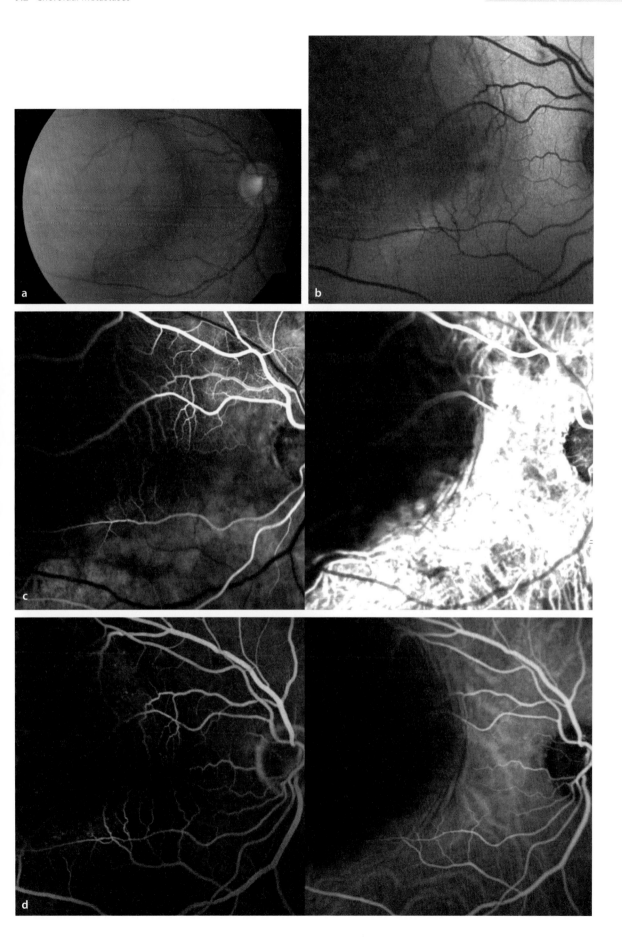

9.3   Choroidal Hemangioma

Choroidal hemangioma is a benign tumor, which is usually located in the posterior pole, and which manifests in the middle decades of life. Fundoscopy shows a red-orange, clearly bordered subretinal prominence. Symptoms arise when the tumor either directly involves the macula or releases subretinal fluid, leading to macular edema. Large choroidal hemangiomas can cause an exudative detachment of the retina. In addition to solitary choroidal hemangiomas, there are diffusely distributed hemangiomas in the setting of the Sturge Weber Syndrome that produce a strikingly red fundus appearance (the so-called »tomato ketchup fundus«).

Fluorescein Angiography

The angiographic appearance of solitary choroidal hemangiomas can be highly varied. Typically, during the early phase, there are irregular areas of hyperfluorescence in the tumor. This hyperfluorescence reflects the filling of vascular spaces within the tumor. This separates the choroidal hemangiomas from other solid, vascular tumors. During the course of an angiogram there is increasing hyperfluorescence with further staining of vascular structures within the tumor. A persistent hyperfluorescence in the late phase can be caused by an accumulation of fluorescein in the vascular spaces of the hemangioma, or by pooling of the dye in subretinal fluid.

ICG Angiography

During ICG angiography the vascular spaces within the tumor are clearly imaged. During the course of the angiogram there is increasing hyperfluorescence corresponding to an accumulation of ICG molecules in the tumor-like vascular segments. After regression of the ICG fluorescence in the surrounding choroid, there remains a persistent ICG fluorescence in the region of the tumor.

◼ Fig. 9.5a–f. A 57 year old patient with a choroidal hemangioma in the left eye. **a** Fundoscopy reveals a subretinal, reddish tumor at the nasal border of the optic disc. **b,c** Fluorescein angiography shows an irregular hyperfluorescence in the tumor at the beginning of the early phase **b**, which increases during the further course of the study **c**. **d** ICG angiography demonstrates vascular segments within the deeper parts of the tumor. **e,f** In the late phase images there is persistent hyperfluorescence in both the fluorescein **e** and the ICG **f** angiograms.

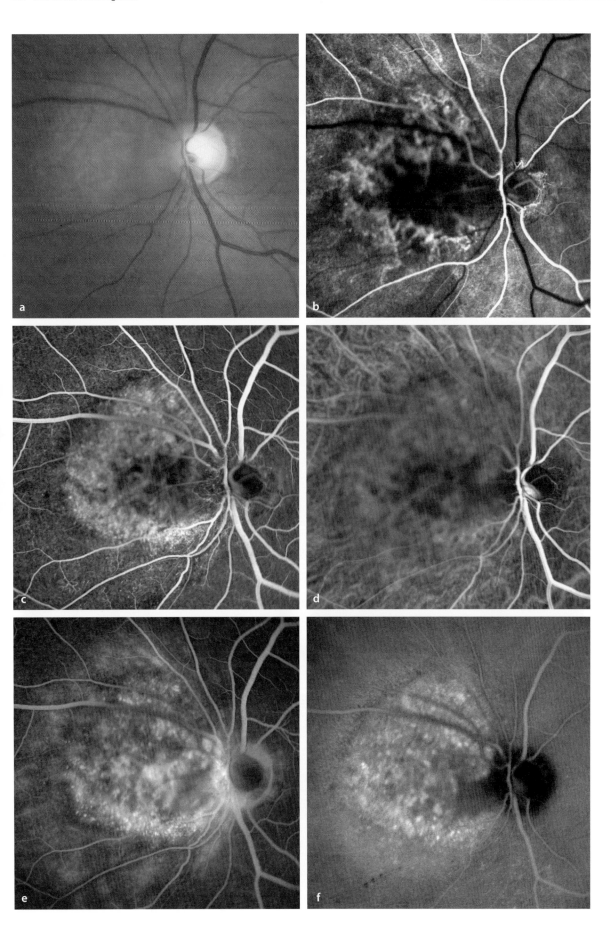

Subject Index

Printing and Binding: Stürtz GmbH, Würzburg